"We do not need to be informed about all the problems involved with being overweight. What we do need are positive messages on how to approach this problem without making it worse and adding more burdens to our lives. Acceptance and commitment therapy (ACT) offers a different message than the usual one. We are encouraged not to struggle in vain, but rather to build a new way of life. This book by Lillis, Dahl, and Weineland is a substantial contribution for persons who are searching for a new way of approaching their weight problems."

—**Gerhard Andersson, PhD**, professor in the department of behavioral sciences and learning at Linköping University, Linköping, Sweden

"In this book, Lillis, Dahl, and Weineland provide a new and refreshing perspective on the struggle to lose weight and adopt a healthy lifestyle. They offer a radically new approach with practical exercises based on acceptance, self-compassion, and behavior change. The book conveys hope, outlines a realistic way of living a valued life, and takes a functional approach toward weight regulation and a healthy lifestyle…. Read this book if you are concerned about your shape and weight: choose life!"

—**Ata Ghaderi**, professor of clinical psychology at Karolinska Institute, Stockholm, Sweden

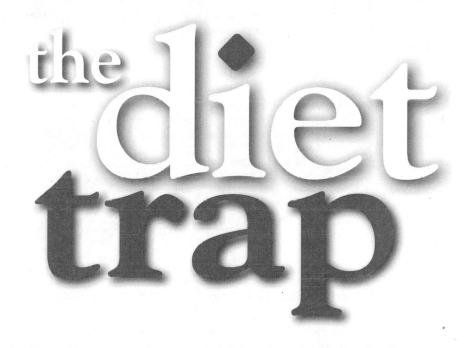

the diet trap

Feed Your Psychological Needs &

End the Weight Loss Struggle Using

Acceptance & Commitment Therapy

JASON LILLIS, PhD | JOANNE DAHL, PhD
SANDRA M. WEINELAND, PhD

New Harbinger Publications, Inc.

Publisher's Note

Distributed in Canada by Raincoast Books

Copyright © 2014 by Jason Lillis, JoAnne Dahl, and Sandra Weineland
New Harbinger Publications, Inc.
5674 Shattuck Avenue
Oakland, CA 94609
www.newharbinger.com

Cover design by Amy Shoup
Acquired by Melissa Kirk
Edited by Jasmine Star

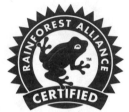

Library of Congress Cataloging-in-Publication Data

Lillis, Jason.
  The diet trap : feed your psychological needs and end the weight loss struggle using acceptance and commitment therapy / Jason Lillis, PhD, JoAnne Dahl, PhD, Sandra M. Weineland, PhD.
      pages cm
  Summary: "The Diet Trap offers proven-effective weight-loss methods based in acceptance and commitment therapy (ACT) to help you change the way you think about food and develop mindful eating habits, so you can ditch the fad diets once and for all, and live a healthier, happier lifestyle"-- Provided by publisher.
  Includes bibliographical references.
  ISBN 978-1-60882-709-1 (pbk.) -- ISBN 978-1-60882-710-7 (pdf e-book) -- ISBN 978-1-60882-711-4 (epub) 1. Reducing diets--Popular works. 2. Weight loss--Alternative treatment--Popular works. 3. Acceptance and commitment therapy. I. Dahl, JoAnne, 1951- II. Weineland, Sandra M. III. Title.
  RM222.2. L47785 2014
  613.2'5--dc23
                          2013036519

Printed in the United States of America

16   15   14

10   9   8   7   6   5   4   3   2   1   First printing

To my mother, for nurturing and
inspiring me on this path.

—Jason Lillis

To my newborn granddaughter, Mildred. May
the spirit of self-compassion underlying this text
be a helping hand in the great journey of life
that you have just embarked on.

—JoAnne Dahl

Dedicated with love to my family:
mum, dad, Robert, and Jeppe.

—Sandra Weineland

Contents

Introduction

If you've tried to lose weight before and struggled to take it off or keep it off, this could be the right book for you. If you've ever beat yourself up, scolded yourself into exercising, blamed yourself for cheating on a diet, or just struggled to find meaning and vitality in the healthy habits you were trying to build, we have an alternative. This book presents a different path to weight loss, and more healthy living in general, through cutting-edge behavior change techniques from acceptance and commitment therapy (Hayes, Strosahl, and Wilson 1999).

The approach in acceptance and commitment therapy (ACT, said as one word) is a compassionate one. We'll teach you how to change your habits humanely, with a focus on getting you in touch with how being healthy fits into a life you really want to have. We'll give you tools for relating to difficult thoughts and feelings differently. We will also focus on doing what works, as opposed to following rigid rules. We want you to love yourself as you make changes, and we'll teach you how to do that. Diet books are often selling a program of sacrifice that will purportedly give you the life you want—eventually. We're selling something different: that you can have the life you want right now, while gradually building healthier habits over time.

One caveat: If you've never tried to lose weight before, there are other, more comprehensive resources that can help you gain the knowledge you need to influence your weight. In this book, we assume that you have a good deal of knowledge about how to lose weight, and that you're struggling to apply that know-how or to sustain changes over time. That's where our methods come in: to teach you how to deal with the barriers that get in the way of applying that knowledge.

We want you to know up front that this book isn't full of dieting advice, step-by-step instructions on how to exercise better, and so on. You'll find no recipes and very little information about nutrition, and we won't be discussing things like the relative worth of margarine versus butter. If you're looking for those things, there are scores of resources that cover those topics, and many of them are very useful. We do have a chapter that covers the basics of weight loss, but it's at the end of the book. Why? We feel that applying weight loss rules doesn't help unless you first fundamentally change your perspective and the way you approach living.

Most of the chapters are structured with a brief client story at the beginning, followed by an easy-to-understand overview of the research findings and ACT approach relevant to topics in the chapter. Then we provide exercises:

some activities to do right away and some to do over time. The ACT approach is experiential. In order to learn the skills, you need to actually do the activities. Understanding concepts is very different from *experiencing* them. For this approach to truly work, you need to engage in the activities and learn from your experiences.

You'll also need to keep a journal while working with the book. Many of the activities require that you do some writing, and we'll usually ask you to use your journal for that. Feel free to use a computer if that works better for you. That said, sometimes you can't beat a good, old-school journal, especially because you can keep it with the book at all times.

The lessons contained in this book build on and complement each other. You may want to read through the book quickly, but to do so, you'd have to skip a lot of the activities. If you want to read the whole thing to get the big picture, go ahead. Plan to read through and do the short activities as you go. Once you finish, start over again, making sure to do all the activities as you read through a second time. Alternatively, you can start by taking each chapter step-by-step. This will be more rewarding, since the skills you learn will naturally grow and build on one another. You can also use this book repeatedly. You may find it helpful to cycle through it multiple times. If you suddenly find that you're off track, come back to it and work through some of the key activities to ground yourself in the core skills and start moving forward again.

We refer to some of the activities as "extended practice exercises." They are just what they sound like: activities meant to be done over longer periods of time, up to a few weeks or even longer. Plan to do a few of these at a time, and introduce new ones when you're ready.

Welcome aboard! We're thrilled that you've chosen to work with this book, and we promise to be honest, compassionate guides throughout your journey. So let's get started!

CHAPTER 1

The Weight Loss Agenda Is the Problem

Because you're reading this book, we're guessing that you're feeling frustrated about your weight. You're probably aware that you need to eat differently or perhaps be more active. You may know approximately how many calories you should be taking in to lose weight, what kinds of foods to eat, and how to track your progress. And yet you still find yourself struggling.

Maybe you've tried to eat less, focused on low-fat or high-protein foods, or relied on prepackaged foods and shakes. These diets probably seemed reasonable. Perhaps you tried to do this on your own or with your partner or a friend, or maybe you attended group meetings. Maybe you joined a gym or hired a personal trainer, or maybe you bought exercise videos or home exercise equipment. If you were to make a list of everything you've tried during all of your years of struggle with weight loss, you'd probably see that at times you were successful in losing weight. In fact, all of this experience might have made you an expert in losing weight. Yet you still find yourself struggling today.

We have some good news for you. If you want to take a new and different approach to losing weight, this book offers an evidenced-based alternative. It will help you take a different perspective on how to live your life, combining the weight loss expertise you already have with a psychological model called acceptance and commitment therapy (ACT, said as one word). Several scientific studies have shown ACT to be effective at promoting weight loss (for example, Lillis et al. 2009) and exercise (for example, Butryn et al. 2011). ACT can help you develop healthy habits that are vital and fulfilling for you. It presents a totally new way to approach weight management, and we believe it can work for you.

We also have some bad news: This book is not a magic pill. Have you ever thought that if you could just get properly motivated, you'd be successful? Or maybe you've thought that if you just found the right recipes, had a little more time, learned the best way to work out, or figured out why you love food so much, it would all fall into place. In fact, picking up this book may be a similar approach. You may be thinking that we've figured out the secret ingredient.

There are no tricks or simple fixes in this book. However, we can offer you an alternative way of living. This isn't just a way to lose weight, but a way to *engage life*—a life that's meaningful, vital, full, and connected; a life that's guided by your inner compass and includes healthy habits as a choice, not as a prison sentence; and, yes, if it truly, deeply matters to you, a life that includes weight control.

If that sounds like something you're willing to explore, then we invite you to join us on a journey. We ask that you come with us on the entire journey, because this isn't the kind of journey you can separate into little pieces. The whole is much greater than the sum of its parts. Also, understand that this is a radically different approach. So if you sometimes feel confused or unsure, or if you sometimes wonder where this is going, know that those feelings are okay and trust that the approach will come together. In fact, let's start the journey by making some room for those feelings and inviting them to come along. Imagine that you're embarking on a long train ride, and those feelings will be sitting in the train alongside you. Might as well invite them, since they're probably coming anyway!

What Science Says About Overweight and Obesity

Before we embark, we think it's important to honor the journey you've already been on. If you've been really hard on yourself, know that you're simply responding to the world as it is. Weight control is no longer the norm in our society. The world we live in promotes obesity, plain and simple. A lot of scientific research has shown this to be the case (French, Story, and Jeffery 2001; Hill and Peters 1998). Although all three of us are science geeks, we promise not to bore you with too much science. However, we do feel it's useful to know a few key things.

First, people experience food as rewarding and pleasurable, some people more so than others, and when you deprive yourself of certain kinds of foods, they may actually become even more rewarding (Saelens and Epstein 1996). If you really love chocolate chip cookies—more than most people do—you'll find them even tastier after not eating them for three months. Not fair! This is especially tough in light of our next point.

Tasty, unhealthy food is inexpensive and easy to get. Manufacturers process food, often by breaking down its healthful components and adding sugar, fat, and salt to maximize taste. They know what we just told you: that people find food rewarding, and by golly, they're going to do their utmost to maximize that pleasure! They also know exactly which foods we find most rewarding, which brings us to our third point.

Eating sugar and fat alters your brain chemistry in a way that makes you want more sugar and fat. Although there's some controversy over this, it does appear that eating fatty and sugary foods changes brain chemistry in ways similar to taking addictive drugs (Volkow and Wise 2005). Obviously, eating pizza doesn't have quite the debilitating effects or extreme dangers of using cocaine. However, eating pizza is likely to lead you to eat more pizza in the future.

So, now we've told you if you eat tasty, unhealthy food, your brain will want more, and we've also told you that if you refrain from eating those foods, later you'll find them to be even tastier. That sounds like a lose-lose proposition!

Of course, this is a simple presentation of the facts, and one that leaves out other important issues, such as eating out, portion sizes, poor urban design, sedentary lifestyles, and so on. In any case, the important thing to note is that our world is now designed to promote steady weight gain. Your only crime is having been born a human being in a society where food is abundant and physical activity is increasingly unnecessary.

EXERCISE: Examining the Unworkable Weight Loss Agenda

We think another factor is important. It has to do with what you've learned about how best to achieve weight loss. Let's explore this a bit. First, circle how many times you've tried to lose weight, even if just for a little while:

0–5 times   5–10 times   10–20 times   Too many to count!

And how many times have you lost weight and gained at least half of it back?

0–5 times   5–10 times   10–20 times   Too many to count!

Now we'll ask you to spend some time writing in your journal. This is the first time, so if you don't have a notebook or journal at hand, stop reading and go get one! Of course, a piece of paper will suffice for now, but don't delay too long.

Imagine that you have a friend who's trying to lose weight. What advice would you give your friend? What would you tell your friend to do? At the top of a page in your journal, write "Advice to a Friend." Then, beneath it, write as much weight loss advice as you can.

***

All done? We're guessing that you wrote very sensible, helpful advice. And yet isn't it the advice you've been given? Isn't at least some of that advice things you've tried or told yourself to do, perhaps over and over again? It might be almost like a song on repeat: *Count your calories. Eat less food. Don't keep cookies in the house. Don't eat at social events. Find tasty low-fat recipes. Exercise more. Get support from friends or family. Stick with it. Don't give up!*

The fact that none of those approaches has worked may make you feel like something is wrong with you. But the problem isn't with you. This kind of advice doesn't work for most people. We think you've been sold a solution that's well-intentioned but ultimately inadequate. That solution, offered by diet companies, the media, and educators alike, is to focus narrowly on your weight and devote your life almost entirely to the task of losing weight, focusing all of your energy and attention on it. The mantra is "Commit, sacrifice, and stay on track!"

We have a radical suggestion: Perhaps the weight loss agenda itself is part of the problem. The usual rules and tips seem to be helpful for losing weight initially, but they don't work in the long term. Narrowly focusing on weight just doesn't work for most people over time.

Take a moment to sit with that idea—that perhaps a singular, narrow focus on weight loss is unlikely to bring the long-term results you want, and that everything you think you need to do, when done solely in the name of weight loss, is a part of an agenda that will ultimately fail. That may sound crazy, but check with your experience— not the rules or beliefs you have in your head, what you've read in books or what you've heard from the media, doctors, or other people. Just check in with your experience. In some deep sense, does your experience tell you this might be true?

For now the question is this: Are you willing to set aside some of your old assumptions about how to lose weight and open up to a new approach that can teach you how to engage life in a way that's more vital and connected to what's important to you? If so, read on. In the sections that follow, we'll examine a number of weight loss myths and explain why the ACT approach is likely to be more effective than old, tried-and-*un*true weight loss strategies.

Missing the Forest for the Trees

Consider this: You probably want weight to be less of an issue in your life. Currently, you may experience your weight as having an influence on your mood, relationships, and self-esteem. Maybe you long for the day when you don't think about your weight very much. Yet supposedly the answer to weight loss is...focusing more on your weight! Could it really be that in order to make weight less a part of your life, you have to devote your life to your weight? Something is fishy here.

Losing weight and maintaining a healthy lifestyle are quite different things. You can lose weight in the short term by becoming hyperfocused on the number on the scale and sheer force of will. Imagine yourself bearing down on the problem with tightly clenched fists, enduring the pain for as long as you can. You can try a few new tricks, eat a very restricted diet, or exercise intensively. But people tend to revert back to old eating habits, abandon exercise programs, and shift their focus to other demands in life. Worse, extreme weight loss efforts can drain the vitality out of a person's life. Have you ever felt beaten down and battered by months and months of dieting? This brings us to the first myth we'd like to bust.

Myth 1: *To achieve lasting weight loss, you have to focus on the task of weight loss at the expense of other priorities until you reach your goal weight.*

To be fair, a narrow focus on weight loss does work for a small percentage of people. They turn their lives over to weight control, and their efforts are successful. However, for the majority of people, this doesn't seem to work. And it's true that you need to have some knowledge about how to influence your weight in order to lose weight. But we're guessing that you already have that knowledge. (If you don't, we'll provide basic information on that topic in chapter 7.) However, we believe that a narrow focus on weight loss is actually part of the problem. And we suggest that you consult your own experience using the following exercise.

EXERCISE: Identifying Problematic Weight Loss Efforts

Open your journal again and write the heading "Problematic Weight Loss Efforts." Then list all of the things you've done in the name of weight loss that seemed to narrow your life or drain it of vitality. Go ahead and make the list now.

***

Looking over your list, you might notice that when you focus only on your weight and the rules you must follow to lose weight, something very important is lost: your life! Rather than empowering your life, these restrictive rules limit it: *Don't do this. Can't do that. Definitely avoid this. Have to stay away from that!* This isn't the substance of a vital, satisfying life or a sustainable path to healthy living.

The more important question is who you want to be as a person. What's important to you? What are you doing in life to pursue what matters most to you? These questions are the key to healthy living. So if you feel like you're grinding through life joylessly and following a set of rules and restrictions that don't enhance your life, it might be time to broaden your perspective and take a look at what you care about and how best to pursue your values in daily life, regardless of what you weigh.

The Fix-Me Trap

The second major reason why a narrow weight loss agenda often doesn't work involves what we call "the fix-me trap." When you struggle with weight loss, do you find yourself feeling frustrated? Again, you probably know what to do to lose weight. So if you know what to do, why haven't you been successful? This often leads to another, deeper question: "What's wrong with me?"

This is a painful question we all deal with at times. When we ask that question, we're usually looking for something fundamentally wrong—something inside of us. You may have had the thought that you need more willpower, don't have enough motivation, lack confidence, like food too much, or are too stressed, sad, or anxious.

EXERCISE: Noticing What Your Mind Says Is Wrong with You

When you've asked yourself, *What's wrong with me?* what kind of answers have you gotten from your mind? We'd like you to explore this now. In your journal, write the heading "What My Mind Says Is Wrong with Me." Take the time now to write the answers to that question that your mind has given you in regard to your weight loss efforts.

✳✳✳

The human mind tends come up with some reliable (and often downright mean) answers to the question "What's wrong with me?" And although these answers are almost always untrue, or perhaps a woefully small piece of a very big picture, they feel real and true all the same. There have probably been times when you believed those explanations for your behavior.

However, we believe that it's important to examine the orientation that lies at the core of this question. If you think there's something wrong inside of you, you're likely to believe that it must be fixed. That last part is really important. Usually the mind presents a solution along with the problem: *If I were just stronger, more confident, more motivated, less attracted to food, better able to handle stress, happier, calmer...* As is probably obvious, the implication is that if the problem were fixed, everything would be different: *I would be successful. Life would be better. I wouldn't be so lonely...* This is what we call the fix-me trap, and it lies at the heart of the second myth.

Myth 2: *There's something wrong inside you, and once you fix it, your life will be better.*

The fix-me trap can get in the way of weight loss, and more importantly, it can interfere with living a vital, satisfying life. When you buy into this trap, you might push the pause button on life. You might say to yourself, *I really need to stop whatever I'm doing and instead focus on changing what's wrong inside me. After I fix that, I can do what's important.*

Have you ever told yourself you'd go to the gym as long as you didn't feel too self-conscious, that you'd initiate sex with your partner only if you felt sexy, or that you'd eat a healthful meal as long as you didn't feel too deprived? How about applying for a job only if there was no chance of feeling rejection, or trying a new hobby or activity only if you felt confident? In all of those scenarios, something about you needed to be fixed or "right" in order for you to do something you probably cared about doing. That's the fix-me trap: requiring thoughts, feelings, bodily sensations (such as cravings), or memories to change or go away in order to live the way you want to. In other words, first you need to think and feel a certain way, then you can do things that matter to you. But is that really how things work? As you might guess, we don't think it is, and that brings us to the next myth.

Myth 3: *You should be able to control what you think and feel.*

Let's do a little thought experiment (based on Hayes, Strosahl, and Wilson 1999). Imagine that we hook you up to the world's most sensitive anxiety-detecting machine. If you feel any anxiety whatsoever, we'll know. Now imagine that we tell you the only thing you need to do is remain completely anxiety-free. You can feel anything else, but not anxiety. Because we want you to do really well at this task, we position a giant wrecking ball twenty feet above you, and if you feel any anxiety, the wrecking ball will fall right on your head.

What do you think would happen? That ball would drop down in less than a second, right? Although people generally believe they can and should be able to control their feelings, emotions often just happen in response to whatever is going on (or isn't going on). If you've got a wrecking ball positioned right above your head, it's likely that you'll feel anxious!

This doesn't happen solely with negative feelings. Here's another thought experiment: Close your eyes and feel the most joy you've ever felt. If you do it right now, we'll give you a million dollars. Ready? Go!

***

How did you do? We bet you'd tell us you did it regardless, because that's a lot of money. But the fact is, we don't have a million dollars, so just assess your reaction honestly: Did you feel pure joy, beyond anything you've ever felt before? What if we told you to feel that joy or the wrecking ball will come down on your head? Can't do it, right?

How about your thoughts? Let's give it a try: For the next two minutes, don't think about your weight or anything related to your weight: how you look, eating, exercising, and so on. Feel free to think about anything else. Ready? Go!

***

Were you able to do it? If not, you aren't alone. Most people find that trying not to think about something, actually causes them to think about it (Wegner et al. 1987).

Then again, perhaps you *were* able to think only about other things. If so, you might have noticed how much work it takes to try to keep your mind occupied and not slip. It can be extremely taxing. Imagine fighting against a thought all day. We all do this sometimes.

But even if you felt you were able to do the task, a paradox arises. Let's say you spent those two minutes thinking about sheep. Sheep have nothing to do with your weight, so that makes sense. But to know that you accomplished the task (not thinking about your weight or anything related to it), you could be sure you did it correctly only by realizing that sheep are...not your weight. Hmm. Something is off here. Like a panicky person frequently checking his or her pulse, you need to think, *Sheep are not my weight*, in order to supposedly not think about weight. In other words, you need to think about your weight to know you're successful in not thinking about it. For this reason, a common ACT saying is "If you can't have it, you've got it." If you want to avoid something, you have to constantly be looking for it to make sure you're avoiding it. This is a problem.

So here we are. Thoughts and feelings seem, at best, hard to control, yet people tend to fall into the fix-me trap, making demands that their thoughts and feelings change so they can live life. Take a look back at your list of things your mind has said were wrong with you and needed to be fixed. Does this really seem like a way forward, fixing all of these things inside you before living life in a vital, meaningful, satisfying way? Your mind might still be saying, *But I do need things to change in order to live that life.* That's okay, but maybe there's another way forward, in weight control and, more importantly, in life.

Weight Loss as a Fix-Me Trap

For many people, weight loss is a version of the fix-me trap: *If I lose weight, then I'll feel confident (sexier, lovable, competent, stronger...). I'll have fewer doubts, fears, and judgments about myself (won't feel ashamed, won't be so down on myself...),* and so on. In other words, losing weight will fix what's going on inside. This can actually work for some people in the short term, and you may have experienced it during some of your weight loss attempts. You might have felt better or noticed that you had more confidence.

If you've experienced this, think back on what happened over the long term. Did you permanently get rid of shame, guilt, sadness, or any of the judgments you have about yourself? Did they go away forever, never to reappear? And if you did notice them coming back, how did that make you feel? Did you want to keep losing weight, or did you begin to feel defeated? How loud did those voices get when you started gaining weight again? How familiar were the self-criticisms? When weight loss becomes mostly about making yourself feel better or think differently, you can be setting yourself up for failure.

Myth 4: *If you lose weight, you'll be happy and think good thoughts.*

The simple truth is that you can't avoid natural and normal human emotions. You are human, after all, and feelings simply come with the gig. Do you remember feeling afraid as a child? Since then, you've been afraid many times. Fear just keeps coming back again and again, kind of like a comet orbiting the sun. It's like that with all emotions. Imagine all of them orbiting around you, sometimes in full view, other times mostly hidden. Sometimes that orbit is quick and you see fear a lot. Sometimes it's slow and lots of time passes between sightings. Some emotions tend to be close by, so you feel them often. Others are more distant and infrequent.

Even if you were to hole up in your room and stay there all day every day, you probably couldn't get rid of unwanted emotions. Something would wear on you: *I'm not doing anything. There's something wrong with me. I'm depressed. I feel lonely.*

On the flip side, if you try to do things in your life that are important, vital, and potentially satisfying, you'll naturally open yourself up to the possibility of pain. (We'll discuss this in detail in chapter 5.) When you open yourself in areas of life that matter to you, like family, relationships, work, and love, unfortunately there will be times when things don't go well. People won't always respond as you wish. You'll have feelings you don't want to have. You'll have thoughts you don't want to have. That's part of the deal. We humans get this amazing chance to live a vital, satisfying life, but the trade-off is that we hurt sometimes. We can't have one without the other.

You may wonder what this has to do with weight loss. If weight loss is about "fixing" you inside (fixing your thoughts, emotions, bodily sensations, and memories), that isn't going to happen. There's no magical weight that will shield you from uncomfortable feelings. You can't summon or banish an emotion on command. So if your weight loss efforts are primarily about fixing your emotions, that's unlikely to work over the long term. Instead, you'll become trapped in an endless loop of trying to fix how you feel.

Likewise, weight loss won't shield you from uncomfortable thoughts. You might be tired of how your judgmental mind always notices and points out flaws, is disgusted with the way you look, and dwells on how things could be different or better. That's understandable, given that magazines flaunt airbrushed pictures of unrealistically thin models, movies are populated with beautiful actors, and so many advertisements are selling the promise that you can be youthful, beautiful, and rich, that everyone will love you, and that your life will be perfect if you just buy their product. It's natural to think that weight loss could help fix some of your thoughts.

Let's do another experiment. Look around the room and pick an object you see—any object. Now see if you can find something to judge about that object. This might seem strange at first, but let yourself go with it. Maybe that trash can is ugly, that cup could be bigger, or the TV could have a clearer picture. Take your time and find a few criticisms of the first object.

Now pick a second object and do the same thing. Then choose a third. Notice how easy this is to do once you get rolling?

The human mind is a judgment machine. That's a big part of what it does. It's constantly categorizing, evaluating, and judging. If you doubt this, quickly answer these questions: Has today been a good or bad day so far? Is this book interesting? What's your favorite TV show? If you had an emergency and could only seek help from one of your neighbors, who would you call?

We bet your mind easily came up with answers to those questions. It did so because it's constantly categorizing, evaluating, and judging. This is an incredibly useful skill. It allows you to take action in life and solve problems both big and small. However, you might have noticed that you are your mind's favorite thing to judge. As with the trash can, cup, or TV, it can find fault after fault after fault.

What does this mean for weight loss? If weight loss is about getting rid of self-judgments or criticisms, that's a lot to ask. Judgment and criticism are a big part of what the human mind does—*all the time*. So even if the specifics change, your mind will continue to remind you of perceived flaws, circumstances that could be different or better in your life, ways you could be doing more, or things you could have that you don't have. Therefore, if weight loss is primarily about fixing your self-judgments or self-criticisms, that strategy is unlikely to work in the long run. Again, you're stuck in the fix-me trap.

Fix Me, Free Me

Have you ever thought how much better life would be if you could just get into a size (fill in the blank)? We know you have a size in mind. Everyone does, and it's pretty much always different from a person's current size. Or perhaps you're thinking you could be firmer here, stronger there, or less round in another area. But let's dig a little deeper into this fix-me trap, in which your life will change once you are thin, athletic, or whatever else is acceptable to your mind. It simply doesn't work that way. We've worked with a lot of clients struggling with their weight, and not once have we had a client whose life was fixed by achieving a certain dress or pant size—never. It may feel good for a short time, but changing your life still requires that you *do something* with your new size. This brings us to the next myth.

Myth 5: *If you lose weight, your life will automatically be better.*

Let's assume for a second that everything up to this point in this chapter so far has been untrue. Let's assume that you could, in fact, think and feel how you wanted, when you wanted, and that you could achieve your perfect weight by fixing yourself inside. Even if this happened, you still wouldn't have the life you wanted—unless you wanted a life that involves sitting in a room all day feeling and thinking great things about yourself. You still have to do the actual living.

This raises some important questions: How do you want to be living? What matters to you? What will you do to actually engage life in the limited time you have on this earth? Changing yourself inside is never a replacement for living. Life is in the living, the doing, the experiencing. It's in the challenges, the ups and the downs, and both the successes and the failures. We humans can get so focused on managing what's going on inside of us that we can lose track of what's really important, yet we all get to choose how to live. There's nothing wrong with achieving and maintaining a healthy weight. In fact, it's a wonderful way to care for yourself and empower a healthy, vital life. But when weight loss is about fixing something that's wrong inside of you, it becomes an unworkable agenda. If this has happened to you, even to a modest degree, you need another way of approaching weight loss that can help you move forward in a sustainable, lasting way. But before you move forward, it's important to take a good look at how you relate to food.

Fix Me, Feed Me

Food is inescapable in our culture. It's a mainstay of celebrations and somber occasions alike. It goes well with entertainment. It seems to be a key part of social gatherings, as well as just hanging around the house. If you have teenage kids, it may be the only thing that gets them to spend time with you. So it isn't surprising that most of us lose track of the fundamental purpose of eating: nourishment.

Food is a means to an end. It gives us energy that allows us to do things in life. But sometimes food becomes a substitute for living, which brings us to the next myth.

Myth 6: *You eat because you're hungry.*

Few of us eat purely to quench hunger. If nourishment were the point of eating, very few of us would be eating hamburgers. Instead, we'd fill up on healthful foods that fuel our bodies optimally. In reality, people use food for a multitude of reasons. For example, if you don't like the way you feel right now, one easy way to try to change that is to eat and experience a physiological pleasure response, especially if you choose sweet, fatty, or salty foods: potato chips, pizza, a burger, cake, cookies, ice cream—the good stuff. You can do it right now...and ten minutes from now...and an hour later. Food is always there. In fact, some fast-food places stay open all night just to make sure a craving doesn't go unsatisfied. (Isn't that nice of them?)

Think about this in light of the fix-me trap: If you don't like what's going on inside you—how you're feeling or what you're thinking—eating can provide comfort or relief. This is sometimes called emotional eating. Have you ever turned to food when you felt stressed? Sugary, salty, and fatty foods activate the pleasure areas of the brain. This helps relieve not just stress, but also anxiety, sadness, boredom, shame, frustration, and sometimes even anger. When you feel uncomfortable, food can help you feel better in the moment. Food delivers.

But as you probably know all too well, while food makes you feel better in the short term, it isn't always good for you in the long run. You might soon feel guilty—perhaps even as you're eating—and begin to experience even more of the emotion you were trying to escape, and heap harsh criticism on yourself as a result. In the longer term, you may experience weight gain, develop physical symptoms, and so on. Efforts to fix what's going on inside tend to make things even worse down the road; and the more you do this, the worse things get over the long term.

We encourage you to practice some self-compassion here. It's natural to want to make yourself feel better. Given the availability of sugary, salty, high-fat foods, it isn't surprising that people reach for them so frequently. Doing so doesn't mean there's something wrong with you. You're simply human. All of us struggle against unwanted thoughts and feelings. Many of us use food to do this—maybe a little, maybe a lot. Recognizing that this struggle is natural and normal is an important first step.

In order to change your relationship to food, you need to understand how food functions for you. If you're using food to influence how you think or feel (less sadness, more joy!), you're probably in a fix-me trap. That should be a red flag. Making the change from using food to influence your emotional state to instead using it primarily for nourishment requires you to take a different approach to your thoughts and feelings, and to living. What we most want to help you do is create a life that's vital, meaningful, and fulfilling. If you can do that, food will come to serve that life, rather than being a substitute for it.

Hating Yourself Thin

If you think back on what triggered most of your diets, you're likely to find various forms of the fix-me trap. You might have looked critically at yourself in the mirror or taken hold of that bulge around your waist and, in disgust, sentenced yourself to a radical diet. Self-loathing can be an effective form of motivation for making radical changes in behavior, but such changes are almost always short-lived, and this approach can be harmful. Punishing yourself in this way is likely to make you feel worse and also drains the vitality from your life. This brings us to the final myth we'll address.

Myth 7: *The more disgusted you are with yourself, the more motivated you'll be to change.*

While it may seem that harsh self-criticism will motivate you to change, the opposite is often true. For people who struggle with weight, disgust and self-judgment often lead to emotional eating (Puhl and Heuer 2009). Yet even as we say this, you might still have the thought that something is wrong with you, and you may believe that thought or even identify with it. That's okay. Please understand that your mind will never stop giving you these thoughts—and that you can choose how to respond to these thoughts. Treating yourself with disdain or disgust won't help you move forward in a sustainable way. You simply cannot hate yourself thin. In fact, this type of motivation typically gets in the way of making changes, as it lands you back in the fix-me trap.

Take a moment to think back to your friend, the one you gave weight loss advice to earlier in the chapter. Let's say your friend was unable to lose weight and keep it off. Is there something wrong with your friend? Is your friend broken? Does he or she need to be fixed in some fundamental way in order to be a valid and whole human being? If nothing about your friend's weight changed, would you still value him or her? The answers to those questions may seem obvious, but when you ask the same questions about yourself, you're likely to get very different answers. For now, just note that and imagine that there might be room for a bit more self-compassion.

The Way Forward

As you're now well aware, we don't think the answer lies in a narrow focus on weight. We're pretty sure it isn't just a matter of trying harder while using the same old strategies. And we know that there's nothing fundamentally wrong with you as a person. We believe that you can achieve what you want in terms of weight loss while also improving your life more broadly. Doing so requires that you take a completely different perspective on what the task is, and we'll help you gain that perspective.

A big part of the approach in this book is getting out of the fix-me trap. We will help you change the way you relate to emotions, thoughts, bodily sensations, memories, and cravings so that your behavior isn't so focused on changing those things, but instead is focused on living the way you want—not after you lose weight, but *right now*. We'll broaden your horizon beyond weight loss and help you figure out how you want to be living in all areas of life. We will also show you how the new skills you'll learn can be applied to the challenge of building healthy habits and, ultimately, losing weight and keeping it off.

In order to do this, you have to take a journey. You have to look at what you're doing not only in terms of eating and exercise, but in your relationships and at work. We'll guide you in clarifying what you deeply care about, how you want to be as a person, and how healthy living will help empower you to pursue a life that's about much more than perceived problems with how you think and feel. Ultimately, you have to fundamentally change how you relate to what goes on inside, letting go of the fruitless struggle to control thoughts and feelings in order to open up to the full range of human experiences and your own potential. That may sound challenging, but we'll help you put it all together into a plan of action and set a new course.

Acceptance and Commitment Therapy

To help empower you to embark on a new course—a path of compassionate, healthy living—we utilize empirically tested techniques from ACT, a newer form of cognitive behavioral therapy. (Cognitive behavioral therapy is the most widely practiced and scientifically sound form of psychotherapy.) Don't be scared off by the "therapy" part; these techniques have also been used in a variety of ways outside of therapy to help people change their behavior, improve their quality of life, and increase their productivity.

In short, ACT assumes that psychological pain (like that which is caused by unwanted thoughts and emotions) is a normal human experience. While our instinct is to struggle with these experiences and try to change how we think and feel, this doesn't always work and often causes us to suffer more, especially when we start putting a lot of effort into avoiding or changing certain thoughts or feelings. ACT teaches people how to let go of the struggle with thoughts and feelings—for example, how to let go of the fix-me trap—and focus more on living well, as opposed to just feeling good.

What if, instead of having to make a craving go away, you could notice that craving with curiosity, try to experience it more fully without giving in to it, and continue to meet your health goals? What if, instead of trying to change how your mind evaluates your body, you could allow your mind to say whatever it wants (*You're fat and ugly!*), notice the judgments simply as transient thoughts, rather than facts, and continue to pursue things that matter, like more fulfilling relationships? What if, instead of pushing away painful emotions such as sadness and trying to avoid them, you could open up to them, honor them as a part of your experience, make room for them as natural human emotions, and carry them with you as you make healthy food choices? These are examples of what we call psychological flexibility: doing things that matter even when psychological barriers are present.

ACT promotes psychological flexibility through mindfulness, acceptance, and values clarification. Mindfulness helps you connect to yourself and whatever is going on in the moment. Acceptance allows you to get unstuck from unhelpful thoughts and let go of efforts to avoid uncomfortable thoughts and emotions. And values clarification reveals what deeply and truly matters to you and how best to pursue that in your life. You'll learn skills in all three of these areas in the rest of this book.

Summary

We have all been sold a narrative, and it goes like this: If you're overweight, there's something wrong with you. You should fix that by losing weight, and when you do, you'll be happy and your life will be better. The way to do that is to focus narrowly on your weight, becoming restrictive and hypervigilant about food, engaging in a lot of exercise for the sake of burning calories, and putting this lifestyle ahead of other priorities.

While this works for many people in the short term, it works for very few people in the long run. This book presents a radically different perspective. Rather than focusing narrowly on the task of weight loss, we'll ask you to look at your life more broadly and make important changes in how you work, play, and relate to people. We want to help you put your energy into living your life fully and consciously, rather than waging war against excess weight and all of the unwanted thoughts and feelings you experience about your weight. We want to help you stop looking for temporary solutions to changing your eating habits and instead examine and radically change your relationship to food.

We'll help you take a compassionate stance toward yourself by developing more mindfulness and acceptance and clarifying your values. We'll also help you recognize, honor, and make room for the full range of human thoughts, feelings, and bodily sensations while also challenging yourself to take steps toward living a more fulfilling, vital life.

Are you ready to start focusing on your whole life and what's deeply important to you, as opposed to just your weight? Are you ready to open up to some of your current and past emotional pain and begin to live life more boldly in the service of getting what you want out of life *and* controlling your weight? Hopefully your answer is yes. If not, that's okay. There's no timetable on saying yes to those questions. The choice is yours to make freely as you progress through this book. Either way, let's begin this journey together.

CHAPTER 2

Self-Compassionate Weight Loss

T he first time Dana could remember feeling disgust and shame about her body was when she was seven years old, in the doctor's office. Her mother had pulled off her dress and the doctor was pinching her skin and shaking his head. From that point on, it seemed like everyone treated Dana as if she had some kind of problem. No matter what she weighed or how she looked, she disliked what she saw in the mirror. Although Dana dated, she felt that most of the guys she went out with were interested in other girls. As a teenager she believed that if she was ever going to have relationships, she had to starve herself, but this never seemed to work. She would starve herself all day long, and when she got home, she would eat uncontrollably. This pattern of starving and bingeing went on for years.

Dana did get married, and she managed to get in shape for her wedding, but soon afterward she lost control again. Her husband started making comments about her weight, which brought up feelings of shame. She tried to compensate by acting sweet and kind even when she didn't want to. The more she pretended, the worse she felt about herself and the more she ate. Dana never left the house to exercise or even be social. She decided that she needed to lose weight first, before she could start living the way she wanted.

Dana's story might be similar to yours, or it might be very different. The details aren't as important as the overall dynamic: Dana fell into a fix-me trap. She knew she was eating too much, making unhealthy food choices, and using food to combat feelings. In response, she harshly sentenced herself to strict behavior changes that were designed not to enhance her life, but rather to fix the emotional pain and self-judgments she was experiencing. The more caught up in fixing herself she got, the less vital and satisfying her life became.

Stigma—The Demotivator

Overweight and obese people experience a great deal of ridicule and sometimes outright discrimination. Our culture seems to believe that if people are overweight, it's their fault; and furthermore, that it's okay to tease them because it may motivate them to lose weight. Rebecca Puhl, a psychologist at Yale University, challenged that notion in a series of ongoing studies.

In one study, she invited women, both overweight and at a healthy weight, to watch a video, supposedly to rate how much they liked new television programs (they didn't know the real purpose of the study). Half of the women saw a neutral video, and the other half saw one depicting an overweight woman in a disparaging manner. Afterward, the women were given a series of questionnaires and access to a spread of food. Interestingly, the healthy-weight women ate the same amount of food regardless of which video they saw, while the overweight women ate three times as many calories after watching the disparaging video (Schvey, Puhl, and Brownell 2011). Mere exposure to weight-based teasing was enough to activate overeating, even though someone else was the target. This flies in the face of the popular notion that "making it uncomfortable" for overweight people will motivate weight loss.

Puhl has conducted a number of other research studies that all show basically the same thing: teasing, ridicule, and discrimination don't motivate people to lose weight; they make it harder to lose weight and actually encourage weight gain (Puhl and Heuer 2009).

Like most people, you've probably started your weight loss efforts from a place of self-dislike. You may have looked at yourself in the mirror, hated what you saw, and decided you had to do something about it. This is completely normal. We all get disgusted with ourselves from time to time, and body shape is an easy target for the judgmental mind. However, losing weight in order to change or get rid of self-loathing thoughts and feelings is a classic fix-me trap: *Losing weight will fix what's going on inside me. I should use the negative thoughts and feelings as motivation.*

But as discussed in chapter 1, you can't hate yourself thin. And in addition to being ineffective, it's a truly unpleasant way to live. If you've tried punishing yourself in this way, you probably found that it not only resulted in quick behavior changes that didn't last long, but also added feelings of shame, inadequacy, or disgust. In other words, it made the self-dislike stronger by adding more assessments of failure. In order to be successful in the long term, you need to build a foundation on something more stable and vital. You need to build it on self-compassion.

The ACT Approach to Change

The fix-me trap is a stance that says, "I'm not worthy, not whole, not valid." In a deep sense, each of us is so much more than the sum of our parts, yet there's a tendency to focus on the parts and which of them need to be fixed.

We believe that if you want to change your life, the best way to do so is to start with radical acceptance of yourself, here and now. If you were to take just one message from this book, we hope it would be to treat yourself with loving-kindness.

We have three main goals in this chapter: to help you see the effects of motivating yourself through self-dislike, to help you connect to a sense of self that promotes self-compassion, and to offer guidance on acting with self-compassion. We want you to approach change with purpose, care, and kindness, rather than beating yourself into change. Once you're able to see and feel the difference between these approaches, you'll begin to discover a new way forward both in weight loss and in life.

It may seem as though we're wandering from our main goal, to promote healthy living. If this concerns you, see if you can make room for the experience of not knowing where all of this is going or how it will come together, and simply immerse yourself in the experience.

EXERCISE: Exploring Self-Dislike, the Enemy of Self-Compassion

We'd like to ask you to take some time to explore why it's so hard to show yourself compassion. In your journal, answer these questions: What are three things you don't like about yourself? And what are two things that would make your life better? Go ahead and do it now.

***

We bet you were able to answer those questions quickly. And, if we were to give you other, similar questions, your mind would gladly supply more answers. (Gee, thanks, mind.) We'll spare you the scientific details, but the human mind has a tendency to create self-dislike and feelings of inadequacy. It's natural and normal. We all dwell on things we don't like about ourselves, painful memories, or times we've failed or been embarrassed. Likewise, we all imagine enjoying circumstances better than our current situation, such as looking different or having more money, a better job, more desirable friends, a better love life, or higher achievements.

We humans can dwell on the negative and dream about alternatives to the point where we can hardly think of anything we like about ourselves and our circumstances. That's why no amount of money can guarantee happiness, and why even the most beautiful people in the world may be disgusted by their bodies. If you have a pet, you might realize that animals don't sit around all day judging their body shape or thinking about how much better life could be. (Yet pet psychiatrists still exist!) It's a uniquely human thing.

EXERCISE: Listing Your Weight Loss Attempts

In your journal, write the heading "My Weight Loss Attempts." Beneath it, list of all the weight loss programs you've tried. As you do so, see if you can identify the specific reasons you began each program, and note any attempt that you made, at least in part, from a place of self-dislike. In other words, if you looked in the mirror one day and thought, *I'm disgusting. I need to do something*, that's an example of self-dislike as motivation. If you ever dieted because you felt shame about your weight, felt criticized by others, or felt you needed to prove someone or yourself wrong, these are all examples of acting from a place of self-dislike.

***

Of course, we all want to feel better, more attractive, sexier, and more confident. And our instinct is to try to achieve that by changing our thoughts and feelings. That's natural. Self-compassion is acknowledging that instinct and honoring it, knowing that you're human, just like everyone else, while also recognizing that this is exactly the instinct that's keeping you from getting where you want to go in life. Buying into the fix-me trap sends you into an endless loop of fighting with your internal experience. Instead, you need a place of strength and stability from which you can act with purpose.

The Enduring You

Who are you? What we're getting at here is who you are in a very deep sense. We might also ask what you are or what defines you. You could spend hours, days, even years thinking about this question and never arrive at a definitive answer. (Indeed, some philosophers have done just that. How did they ever pay the bills?)

Typically, people begin answering those questions by listing attributes, like gender, race, ethnicity, age, height, and weight; roles, such as father, mother, son, daughter, friend, worker, or lover; perceived characteristics, such as smart, strong, emotional, or happy; and psychological aspects, such as their beliefs, dreams, desires, values, struggles, and so on. And yet each descriptor or characteristic is only a small piece of the whole.

The following exercise (inspired in part by Hayes, Strosahl, and Wilson 1999) will help you begin to discover a sense of self that isn't defined by its parts. We call this sense of self the "enduring you."

EXERCISE: Exploring the Enduring You

In your journal, start a new section entitled "The Enduring Me." Then call to mind something you experienced last year, preferably something relatively neutral. When you have something in mind, write about it, describing what happened, who was there, what you saw and heard, and everything you took in through your senses. Be as detailed as possible. Also describe thoughts you had, emotions you felt, and so on. Again, be as detailed as possible. Spend at least a few minutes on this.

***

When you're done, consider the following questions: Who saw what you saw? Who felt the emotions you felt and thought what you thought? Who smelled what you smelled and touched what you touched? And who observed every bit of what happened there? You, of course, but which you? The tall person, the parent, the smart person? That can't be it.

In some deeper sense, there's a you that was there then, just as you are here now. Connect to that. You were there then, and you are here now. Even though lots of things have changed, you're still you. You have observed everything that's happened, witnessed it, experienced it. You've been there the whole time. Although many things in your life have changed since last year, in some deep sense you are the same "you" that you were back then. That part of you that goes on, unchanged, is what we call the enduring you.

Now think of something you experienced as a child. When you have something in mind, write about it in the same way: what happened, who was there, everything you took in through your senses, and your thoughts and feelings. Again, be as descriptive as possible and spend at least a few minutes on this.

***

Now see if you can notice that the enduring you was present then, just as it is now. In some deep sense, you've been you your whole life. This essence of you, the enduring you, was there to witness everything that happened to you as a child, everything you did, felt, thought, saw, heard, smelled, touched, and tasted. The enduring you was there, experiencing it all, and yet, in some sense, it has remained completely unchanged by those experiences. You were there then and are here now. Although aspects of you and your behavior have changed, the enduring you remains, watching, observing, and experiencing everything you watch, observe, and experience.

Now think of a time when you felt emotional pain that was somehow related to your weight, from any time in your life. Again, write a detailed description of what happened, who was there, everything you took in through your senses, and your thoughts and feelings. Spend at least a few minutes writing about this.

***

Now notice that time has passed and your body has changed. You were there then and are here now. Perhaps you weigh more or less, but the enduring you has remained the same. The same you was there during this incident, feeling what you felt, thinking what you thought, seeing what you saw. The enduring you was there during the painful time you just described, in your childhood, and it was there a year ago, and it is still here. You have been you for your entire life. And through it all, through all the joy, pain, growing, illness, and changes, you are still you.

Draw a timeline in your journal and fill in some of the major milestones of your life. Create a visual, sequential representation of some of the major changes and accomplishments in your life. Take some time to complete your timeline right now.

***

Now review your timeline and see if you can connect with the fact that, in some fundamental way, at every step along the journey you were there, experiencing everything. The enduring you has been around the entire time, witnessing everything, even as aspects of you changed dramatically.

The Enduring You Doesn't Need Fixing

The word "enduring" means lasting and durable. The enduring you has certainly lasted, having been there your whole life, and is certainly durable, remaining unchanged no matter what happened to you, able to continuously observe, witness, and experience whatever happens. And it continues to be there, experiencing all that you're experiencing right now as you read this book. Again, this doesn't mean your attitudes, beliefs, thoughts, feelings, and behavior haven't changed. In fact, they probably have changed—and quite frequently. However, through it all there's an essence of you that's stable and enduring, no matter what.

This can be comforting. Through everything, no matter what happens, a part of you—the enduring you—remains intact, consistent, and stable. No amount of weight gain can change the enduring you. No emotional experience, criticism from others, or self-judgment can change it. No matter what, the enduring you will still be there, seeing all that you see, experiencing all that you experience, and grounding you.

From this perspective, the fix-me agenda becomes less important. If, in a deep sense, you are much more than your feelings and thoughts, perhaps your feelings and thoughts don't have to be a certain way for you to live your life as you want to. Maybe they don't need to be fixed for you to be fundamentally okay and valid as a person.

Think about your body. It has changed so much. You used to be a tiny baby, and now you're fully grown. Your weight has changed; in fact, it's changing slightly every second you're alive. Sometimes you've been bigger, other times smaller. And yet in some deep sense, the enduring you hasn't changed. Would you say that when you were smaller you weren't you? Of course not. You've been you your whole life. That continuity is the enduring you.

The cells inside your body are constantly dying and regenerating. Most of the cells you were born with are dead. Fat cells in particular die and regenerate quickly. There are virtually no fat cells in your body that were there ten years ago. So, while you have a body with cells, organs, fluids, and so on, you can't be simply your body. You're something more than that—something stable and enduring.

Try to identify a feeling you're having right now, even if it's just contentment, boredom, or curiousity. Whatever that feeling may be, is this the first time you've felt that feeling? Probably not. Think of other times you've felt this feeling. Get specific and identify two or three instances.

Feelings are transient; they come and go. Sometimes you're sad, other times happy, sometimes bored, other times stressed, sometimes content, other times curious, sometimes anxious, other times guilty, and so on. So while you experience feelings, you must be much more than just your feelings. In some sense, the enduring you has been around all along, feeling everything that you've felt as the emotions come and go. It has witnessed and experienced all of your feelings, and yet in some fundamental way, it remains unchanged by them. After all, you are no more "you" now than you've been in the past.

Identify one belief you have now that you didn't have when you were younger. When your belief changed, did you become a different person? Of course not. So while you have feelings, thoughts, beliefs, and sensations, you can't be simply your feelings, thoughts, beliefs, and sensations. The essence of you is much more than these experiences.

It's as if all of these experiences are the content of your life, and you, the enduring you, are the container. You contain all of your experiences and always have room for more. You're intimately in contact with all of your experiences and yet are something more than them. The container is unaffected by the changes and all of the ups and downs, and it will continue to be there, holding everything, as long as you're alive.

EXERCISE: Visualizing the Enduring You

Take some time to imagine what your container looks like. Then draw a picture of it in your journal. You might want to extend the drawing across two pages so you have more room. In that container, depict some of the experiences of your life. For example, you could portray thoughts, feelings, memories, roles, attributes, experiences—anything you want. Represent these things with objects of various sizes. As you do this, notice that no matter what you put inside, the container remains the same. Go ahead and make the drawing now.

If the essence of you, the enduring you, is the container, you don't need to be so invested in what shows up inside of it. That container is big enough and the enduring you strong enough to hold it all. You can also notice a distinction between you and what you contain. In other words, there's you, and there's the stuff you experience. The stuff comes and goes. You endure.

It's like a movie screen. Sometimes a comedy is playing, other times a drama, sometimes a documentary, other times a romance, sometimes a scary movie, other times an adventure flick, and so on. As the movies play, you may notice dramatic emotional swings and thoughts coming, going, and bouncing all over the place. After a truly scary movie, you may feel terrified; after a tragedy, broken. The movies change, over and over. Notice that as they do, the screen remains the same. You are the screen—the context in which all the drama, joy, comedy, and fear unfold. Through it all, the enduring you remains a constant, always witnessing all that's happening, but in some deep way unchanged, stable, steady, perpetual, and dependable.

What Is Self-Compassion?

Taking the perspective of the enduring you might make it easier to treat yourself with self-compassion. You may be able to recognize that you are, in fact, whole and valid just as you are. The internal stuff you've been fighting with isn't you anyway, so you can honor it simply as part of your experience. This is a big part of self-compassion.

An effective way to begin practicing self-compassion is to treat yourself with loving-kindness: to be caring toward yourself, especially when you're suffering. This may seem simple, but it can be hard to do. It involves noticing when judgmental thoughts are present and you find the pull to beat yourself up, and acting instead with kindness. Think of acting toward yourself as you might toward a cherished loved one who's struggling.

Another key to self-compassion is opening up to your pain. You may have a myriad of thoughts, feelings, and memories related to being overweight. Self-compassion means being aware of what's going on inside you, being moved by your own suffering, and showing empathy toward yourself and your history. This is easier when you take the perspective of the enduring you. Those experiences are the stuff of your life, and the enduring you is spacious enough to contain all of them and still move forward.

A final key to self-compassion is to behave in ways that matter to you. One of the best ways to practice self-compassion is by doing things that you find worthwhile: engaging in stimulating and vital activities, seeking and fostering connections with others, taking care of yourself physically and emotionally—whatever matters to you.

The next two exercises will aid you in developing self-compassion. The first fosters gratitude for your body. The second is a way of exploring your values and how you want to live your life.

EXERCISE: Extending Gratitude to Your Body

Read through this exercise in its entirety before doing it, and find a quiet place to practice where you won't be disturbed.

Take a minute to get in touch with yourself. Notice how you're sitting and what it feels like to be sitting. Become present with yourself and observe how your body takes care of you. Your body seems to know exactly what you need, and it tries to provide what you need to be more balanced. See if you can just notice the wisdom of your body—that whatever you do, however you behave, your body accepts things the way they are and does its best to work toward a healthy balance.

See if you can observe your heartbeat, perhaps putting your hand gently on the left side of your chest. Imagine how this heart of yours has been with you from the beginning, and how it has served you, day and night, through all the years of your life. This heart of yours has pumped more blood when you needed to run or climb stairs and pumped less when you sat still. Your heart has never judged you harshly; rather, it has accepted and served you in whatever ways you demanded. Perhaps you'd like to take a moment and thank your heart for its nonjudgmental way of serving you.

Can you feel your stomach or parts of your digestive tract? You might feel these organs at work, sorting out what you've been eating into what your body can use right now, what to discard, and what to store for later. Your digestive tract has put up with all your dieting efforts, no matter how extreme, and hasn't judged you; rather, it has done its best to make do with what you've provided. Take a moment to show appreciation to your digestive tract for the compassionate way it has served you all your life.

Now focus on your brain. It's an incredible marvel, composed of literally billions of neurons firing as it organizes everything you do: from circulating necessary fluids throughout your body, to sending the information required to move your limbs, as well as thinking, problem solving, and so on. Pause for a moment and extend gratitude toward your brain. Your brain serves you in the best way it can and hasn't asked for anything in return. Allow yourself to notice and appreciate the enormity of the job your brain has been given, and as you do, see if you can show it some appreciation.

Now take a moment to fully experience what acts of self-compassion feel like in your body. Take a minute to simply experience the compassion you've created before you change gears and return to reading this book or go on to other activities.

Self-compassion may seem like a simple concept, but it can be hard to practice. You may have noticed, even in this exercise, that you had difficulty showing gratitude toward your body. It often seems easier to extend empathy and compassion to others than to oneself. Fortunately, the behaviors and attitudes involved in compassion for others are the same as those needed for self-compassion—for example, active listening, sensitivity to wants and needs, and a willingness to act on these signals. The trick is to turn these well-practiced skills toward yourself.

EXERCISE: Creating a Memorial to Painful Memories

In your journal, and start a new section entitled "Memory Memorial." Call to mind a difficult memory related to your weight. Perhaps you've experienced ridicule, discrimination, or shame related to your weight or shape at some point in your life. This is a memory of yours, something you experienced. It's one of the items in your container. Take a few minutes to write briefly about what happened and how you responded to it.

***

We humans have a tendency to want to make unhappy memories go away, and we'll go to great lengths to avoid having them pop up for fear of having to look at them again and again. However, in this exercise, we ask that you *honor* this difficult memory.

Throughout your life, you've had lots of experiences that turned into unpleasant memories. And yet here you are today, enduring. Think about your container, with all of the stuff inside, and imagine that there's a memorial in one particular spot in your container. This particular memorial is meant to honor all of your painful memories and to serve as a symbol of the fact that, through all of the pain, you have endured. You continue. What might this memorial look like? Think of a type of memorial that you like, be it a statue, sculpture, fountain, or park. Then, in your journal or on a piece of paper, draw a detailed picture of the memorial. What is the setting like? Is it in a field, near water, or in a building? Now imagine etching the particular weight-related memory you identified into your memorial.

A memorial is an object that serves as a remembrance of something. Memorials usually aren't meant to make us feel happy; rather, they serve to honor the past and keep memories alive. From time to time, you'll pass by this memorial and honor your journey and perseverance. Other times there will be new memories to etch. Ignoring the memorial or trying to pretend it's not there is a form of self-dislike. It's like saying that there's something wrong with a piece of your history and the memory you now have because of it. It's the opposite of self-compassion.

So how do you honor this memory? You can start by acknowledging that it happened and that whatever you did in response was what you were able to do at the time. Allow yourself to make peace with this memory. Time has passed, and you endure. Recognize that it's okay to feel what you feel, and open up to that feeling fully with the knowledge that the enduring you can handle anything you feel.

You can also commit to doing something in service of this memory. Pain and loss have a way of revealing what matters.

EXTENDED PRACTICE EXERCISE: Doing What Matters

One of the best ways to practice self-compassion is by doing the things that give you a sense of meaning and vitality in life. Today—right now—identify one thing that matters to you, one important thing you could do to make your day more meaningful and satisfying Note that this shouldn't be a fix-me behavior. In other words, if you think, *I want to let myself eat some ice cream because it will taste good and make me feel better,* you're definitely falling into a fix-me trap. The goal of the behavior shouldn't be "feeling better" by getting rid of difficult internal experiences; rather, it should be doing something meaningful and satisfying—something that you'll later experience as being worth your time, regardless of how it felt while doing it. Examples include reaching out to a friend or family member, engaging in a hobby or activity that you haven't done in a while, or pursuing an important vocational skill or opportunity. These are acts of self-compassion because they build vitality and strengthen the awareness that you can always do important things, regardless of what's going on—inside you or outside.

Once you've identified a meaningful act you can do today, write it in your journal, then check back at the end of the day to make sure you did it. When you check back, take a few minutes to write about your experience of doing this activity and what it meant to you. This is an exercise you could do every day. Try it for a week and then continue to do it as often as you find helpful.

Self-Compassion Through Mindful Awareness

Mindfulness is the ability to connect to your experience in the present moment, which may include anything you sense (anything you touch, smell, taste, see, or hear), your thoughts, or your feelings. Mindfulness is also a way to focus your attention. It can help you remember information, learn more quickly, and bring awareness to important things, like goals or potential solutions to problems.

Importantly, mindfulness is also inherently self-compassionate. Through mindfulness practice you can tune in to your body without judgment. As you become a better observer of your experiences, you can respond in more compassionate ways. Tuning in to what's going on inside, as opposed to pushing it away, is the first step in changing how you relate to your experiences. It also helps build a more compassionate way of relating to sensations, thoughts, and feelings.

The purpose of mindfulness is to be aware of what's going on around you and inside you with curiosity and openness. It's about slowing things down and connecting with your experience through questions like these: *How do I feel? What's going on with me? What are my needs? What's an important thing I want to accomplish today? Am I doing things that matter to me? Am I treating other people in a loving, kind way? Am I treating myself in a loving, kind way?*

The next three exercises will teach you some very basic mindfulness skills, which we'll build on in later chapters. The goal is to build a foundation by training your focus and attention.

EXERCISE: Tuning In

Mindfulness may sound complicated or abstract. It's actually a simple skill aimed at purposely focusing your attention, as this exercise demonstrates.

Start by looking around the room. Identify ten things you see and name them.

Next, for one minute focus on the sounds you hear. Even if you're in a "quiet" room, see if you can notice that there are many sounds.

Next, focus your attention on your body for one minute. Notice if you're relaxed or tense, tired or energetic, and so on. Simply observe how your body feels, with curiosity, for one full minute.

***

You're already on your way to being a mindfulness master! One of the keys to mindfulness is to take the stance of an observer. Your job is to open up to and simply observe or notice whatever shows up, and then focus on specific parts of your experience without getting caught up in them.

EXTENDED PRACTICE EXERCISE: Practicing Mindful Breathing

In this exercise, you'll practice noticing your breathing. This is a core mindfulness skill. The point isn't to influence your breath or what's happening inside you, but rather to gently direct your attention to the breath and observe your experience as it unfolds. This is an important distinction. Mindfulness means becoming a master observer of everything that happens to you and within you. If you get caught up in trying to change what's going on, you've moved out of mindfulness. We recommend that you read through the entire exercise before doing it. Initially, it's best to find a quiet place to practice where you won't be disturbed.

Sit quietly and breathe through your nose, focusing your attention on the area just below the tip of your nose and above your lip. See if you can maintain your attention on this area just below your nose. See if you can feel the difference between your inhalation and exhalation in this area. See if you can feel the difference in temperature here as you breathe in and breathe out. If you can't feel your breaths, try breathing slightly harder until you can feel the temperature of your breath. As soon as you can feel your breathing on your skin, breathe normally again. See if you can keep your attention on this area for ten slow breaths, in and out.

Next, focus your attention on the point at which the air enters and then exits your body, again focusing your attention on the inhalation and exhalation at this point. See if you can keep your attention on this area for ten slow breaths, in and out.

Next, shift your attention to the rise and fall of your torso. As air fills your lungs, your torso expands, and as it leaves your lungs, your torso falls. See if you can focus your attention on the ebb and flow of this expansion and contraction of your torso. Do this for at least ten slow breaths, in and out.

Throughout this practice, you may notice your attention wandering to other things: thoughts about what you need to do later, judgments about how you're doing the exercise, and so on. That's fine. Each time, just gently bring your attention back to the task.

After focusing on your breath in your torso, circle back and go through the exercise again, focusing first on the area just below the tip of your nose, then on the point where the air enters and exits, then on your torso. Continue to practice for at least five minutes.

Mindfulness takes practice, and like muscle strength it must be built up over time and through repetition. Practicing mindfulness of the breath will help you sharpen your awareness. Try to practice this skill daily for at least a week, and then continue to practice it as often as you find helpful.

EXTENDED PRACTICE EXERCISE: Tuning In to the Body

In this exercise, you'll spend some time tuning in to your body. This can be more difficult, because many people tend to notice all kinds of thoughts and feelings associated with the body. However, this makes it the perfect place to practice mindfulness!

We recommend that you read through the entire exercise before doing it, and that you find a quiet place to practice where you won't be disturbed. For the ten minutes of the exercise, allow yourself to be guided simply by the awareness of what's happening in your body. Take a self-compassionate stance, and observe from the perspective of the enduring you. Simply watch, witness, and describe your experience. If you notice judgments or feelings, note them and then gently direct your attention back to your body and the sensations in your body.

Close your eyes and begin by practicing mindfulness of the breath for at least two minutes.

Next, move your attention to the top of your head. Use your attention like a sensitive instrument and gently scan back and forth over the couple of inches on the top of your head, noticing whatever you feel. Don't look for or expect certain sensations; simply notice whatever sensations are actually there.

When you're able to sense physical sensations on the top of your head, turn your attention to other parts of your body. Move your attention to any part of your body and see if you can detect the unique physical sensations from that particular part of the body. For example, you may notice tension, tightness, warmth, relaxation, movement, lack of movement, heaviness, lightness, smoothness, or rhythms. Your job is to simply observe and describe what you experience. You might point your awareness to your shoulders, noticing their position, any tension or fatigue, then move to your chest, arms, legs, feet, toes, and so on, noticing sensations in the same way. Try to see how small an area you can sense. This will help sharpen your attention.

Practice observing physical sensations in various parts of your body for at least ten minutes. As you practice, you may notice your attention wandering to other things: thoughts about what you need to do later, worries about things that have happened, judgments about how you're doing the exercise, and so on. That's fine. Each time just gently bring your attention back to mindfulness of the body.

***

What places did you choose to focus on? For example, did you tune in to the top of your head, your eyes, or your shoulder muscles? What sensations did you feel? Perhaps you felt warmth, pulsation, or crawling sensations. Tuning in can be sometimes interesting, sometimes uncomfortable, and frequently hard. But as you become more in tune with your body, you can make choices about how to respond to what's going on inside you. As you allow yourself to observe what's going on inside you more often, you'll notice a natural shift toward more self-compassion and openness.

As with mindful breathing, we recommend practicing this skill daily for at least a week. Practicing mindfulness of both the body and the breath is an important foundation for the work you'll do with this book. We'll build on these skills as we teach you how to relate to your thoughts and feelings differently and help you focus on what matters to you so you can chart a new course in life. This course starts with taking a simple, compassionate stance, affirming that whatever you sense, feel, and think is okay.

Weight Loss Revisited

Take a moment now to begin charting a new course. From the perspective of the enduring you, thoughts are simply that—thoughts—not absolute truths. You can mindfully observe and describe them, letting them be as they are. Feelings are simply that—feelings—transient states that come and go throughout life. You can make room for them to ebb and flow naturally. Memories are simply that—memories, snapshots of life experiences. You can mindfully notice their historical nature and separate that from what's happening right now.

From this perspective you can let go of the fix-me trap and focus on the bigger picture of how you want to live. But this may raise some questions: What do you want to do? What would be a more compassionate, vital course for healthy living?

EXERCISE: Identifying Self-Compassionate Reasons to Live a Healthier Lifestyle

Take a moment now to generate a list of reasons to live a healthier lifestyle, reasons that are consistent with self-compassion. Imagine what a more healthful lifestyle will provide to your body and allow you to do in your life. Here's a hint: If anything you write has to do with thinking or feeling differently because you've lost weight, you're off track and have wandered into fix-me land. Circle back and think of ways healthy living can empower you to live your life with purpose and vitality. Does it enable you to engage with family and friends more or more authentically? Does it help you do activities that you currently find difficult? Does it allow you to set an example for others or help you be more nurturing or loving? In your journal, write the heading "Self-Compassionate Reasons to Adopt a Healthier Lifestyle," then list the reasons that fit best for you. If you find this difficult, come back to this exercise after you've worked through a few more chapters.

Summary

This chapter helped you explore self-compassion and how this stance differs from being motivated by self-dislike. Connecting to a stable sense of self, what we call the enduring you, is important in avoiding the fix-me trap. From this perspective, acts of self-compassion are more natural. Acting with self-compassion can lead to lasting changes in behavior, whereas changes spurred by the fix-me mentality tend to be short-term at best. The next few chapters will focus on skills for dealing more compassionately and effectively with the thoughts and feelings that pull you into the fix-me trap.

CHAPTER 3

Don't Change Your Thoughts, Change Your Behavior

Gina struggled to lose weight. As a working mother of three, she felt very busy. She did well when she started diets, but over time she'd feel that her thoughts betrayed her. After the kids went to bed, she felt like the cupboards were talking to her. Of course, the cupboards weren't actually talking to her (at least, we hope not!), but she was having a lot of intrusive thoughts about food, wanting to snack, craving desserts, and so on. These thoughts always came when life quieted down, if just for a few moments. She found herself struggling with them, and it seemed that the only way to make them go away was to give in and eat something.

When she was doing well, Gina noticed more thoughts along the lines of *You got this; don't worry* or *You can have some of that; it won't hurt* or *You're doing so well; you deserve this!* At first she'd ignore these thoughts, but over time they wore her down, and she'd slip back into old eating habits. This led to other thoughts, now more like *You blew it* or *You'll never succeed* or *You're weak and disgusting.* These thoughts often led her to quit her diet and hit rock bottom.

EXERCISE: Noticing the Constant Stream of Thoughts

Our minds produce thoughts—lots of them, and constantly. If you just tune in and listen to your mind, you can almost hear the engine running. Memories, judgments, endless to-do lists, worries, plans, songs, random ideas, rules about what to do and what not to do, and on and on. Take a minute now and try to listen to your thoughts. Just notice all of the activity going on in your mind. Take your journal out and, on a new page, write down every thought you're having, as quickly as you can, for three minutes. Feel free to use shorthand or single words rather than full sentences. If you have thoughts like *Am I doing this right?* or *I have no thoughts*, notice that those are thoughts too and write them down. Go ahead and do it now.

***

That's a lot of thoughts, right? We live in a constant stream of them, our minds generating thought after thought after thought. We seldom see this process, and instead just live inside the endless stream of thoughts our minds produce.

Thoughts can be very powerful. They can push and pull us around. We can become so invested in not having certain thoughts, such as *I'm weak*, that we avoid doing something important, such as dieting, for fear of failure. We may become so invested in having a certain thought, such as *I'm a good person*, that we might work endlessly at something, such as doing things for others, at the expense of our own life. When we play the "control our thoughts" game, we frequently lose. We can get off track and out of touch with what's important and what works. This is a fix-me trap in relation to thoughts. When we do things mostly to influence what we think, we've fallen into the trap.

The Pesky White Bear

If we don't like a thought, it makes sense to get rid of it or replace it with something we do like. But how well does this work? Psychologist Daniel Wegner spent years studying thought suppression. He wanted to know what happens when we try to make thoughts go away, so he did a series of experiments, including his now famous white bear study, in which he simply asked participants to try to think about anything but a white bear. That may seem odd, since most people don't think of a white bear very often, but that was the point. What Wegner and his colleagues found was that, in general, suppressing or getting rid of a thought isn't that easy (Wegner et al. 1987). Few people were truly successful at doing it. More important, however, was the finding that people who were successful at suppressing those thoughts experienced a rebound effect: later, they had many more thoughts about a white bear, and those thoughts felt much stronger. Suppression, it seemed, had the opposite effect of what was intended.

Think about that for a moment. How often have you told yourself not to think about something? How often have you tried to replace a negative thought with a positive one? We all do this. Society offers many messages that we should be able to do this ("Just think happy thoughts," or "Mind over matter"). So we probably shouldn't be surprised that we feel bad when we can't control our thoughts, as many of us do. This seems a lot like a fix-me trap. Perhaps there's an alternative.

The ACT Approach

We suggest you sidestep the fix-me trap by changing your relationship to your thoughts without trying to change the actual thoughts. For example, let's say you struggle with the thought *I'm disgusting.* You could try to control that by never getting in situations that would give rise to that thought, such as sex with your partner, stepping on the scale, or going to the gym. However, if you value intimacy and health, this strategy won't be good for you, especially in the long run.

If instead you can change your relationship to the thought *I'm disgusting* and experience it as a thought and nothing more, then it won't matter as much if you have that thought while pursuing what matters to you. You could let go of controlling that thought and initiate intimacy, step on the scale, or go to the gym, knowing full well that the thought *I'm disgusting* is likely to show up. In a sense, you're allowing that thought to be there without being so attached to the content of the thought or its meaning. To do that, it's helpful to start seeing your thoughts from a radically different perspective.

To see your thoughts from a different perspective, you first have to get better at noticing the process of thinking. That may sound strange, but bear with us here. To change your relationship to your thoughts, you need to become more aware that you're having thoughts. Then you can step out of the constant stream of thoughts and practice looking at them. When you get some distance from your thoughts, you can experience them with less attachment or struggle. Because few people are taught how to do this, it will probably take a lot of practice. The rest of this chapter provides exercises and other guidance on experiencing your thoughts differently so that you can focus more on healthy living, even when unhelpful thoughts show up.

Hello, Mind!

The longest relationship you'll have in your life is the relationship you have with your mind. It's been there for as long as you can remember, and it will be there until your death. So we want to take this opportunity to do a proper introduction. You, Mind... Mind, you... Good, now that we've done that, we're going to say something your mind won't like: Your mind isn't always your friend! There, we said it. It's not that your mind has bad intentions; it's just that its methods aren't always beneficial. But we're getting ahead of ourselves.

You may notice that your mind never shuts up. Even when you're asleep, it dreams, often spinning out some pretty weird stuff. First thing in the morning it starts reminding you of all the things you have to do that day. And when you really need to relax? Ha! Usually that's when it pumps up the volume (*You have so much to do!*). On it goes, constantly chattering, commenting on everything, worrying, reminding you of stuff, worrying about imagined future scenarios. Like the Energizer Bunny, it keeps going and going.

When it comes to weight loss, your mind can be like the world's worst motivational speaker. It thinks it's doing you a favor. It thinks it's helping you live your life. In fact, it's often doing quite the opposite. Our minds evolved to keep us out of danger, so they usually focus on the negative, like past hurts and failures, what isn't going well right now, and what could go wrong in the future: *Remember when they laughed at you?... Everyone thinks you're fat and ugly... Nobody is going to take you seriously... You're going to die alone!* These kinds of reminders are supposed to motivate you to change and live a healthier, fuller life. And for a few people, this does actually help them change. Most of us, however, aren't motivated by this nonsense.

In fact, research shows that these kinds of stigmatizing thoughts drive people to do the very things they're trying not to do (Puhl and Heuer 2010). Such thoughts push us to seek comfort in an attempt to avoid feeling bad. A good way to keep from feeling bad in the short term is by avoiding hard stuff, like working out in a gym with other people around, and a great way to feel better in the short term is, of course, that old friend: eating. This is just another way of getting stuck in the fix-me trap, trying to change what's going on inside at the expense of doing things that matter.

EXERCISE: Seeing Your Mind as a Misguided Motivational Speaker

Take out your journal and write the heading "My Mind's Worst Motivational Speech." Then take at least five minutes to write your mind's most misguided motivational speech. Be sure to use all of your mind's greatest motivational hits—for example, *You're disgusting. Who would ever want to be with you?* Go ahead and write it now.

***

Now read that speech out loud, picturing your mind as a cartoon character or news personality whom you don't find credible. You could choose Daffy Duck, Mickey Mouse, Geraldo Rivera, George Bush, Bill Clinton—whoever fits the bill for you. Try it with at least two different characters. Go ahead and do it now.

***

How was that experience? It probably felt a little strange, but you may also have found it hard to take the speech so seriously. This is just a brief example of what we mean by changing your relationship to your thoughts. Your mind has probably told you many of the things in that speech over and over again. And have no doubt, it will do so again in the future. When you're stuck in your thoughts, those words seem true, important, and real. It feels as though, in order to live the way you want to, you first have to fix or change those thoughts, do things to make them go away, or, better yet, prove them wrong.

But if you become aware that you're thinking, that your mind is producing thoughts, then you can notice that this is just your mind doing its thing. It's speech time again, and you're the captive audience. If you can picture the thoughts coming from somewhere or someone, suddenly there's a little breathing room between you and what your mind is saying.

Maybe you don't need to struggle with, buy into, or act on those thoughts. Maybe they just play like a broken record, repeating bad advice from a well-meaning but seriously misguided motivational speaker. Maybe that speech isn't going to help you get where you want to go.

If it isn't, do you need the speech to change? Do you need the "right" motivational speech from your mind? Probably not. Maybe you can just let your mind give its speech and choose to do things that matter to you while the speech drones on in the background.

EXERCISE: Understanding Where Thoughts Come From

In this exercise, we'll take a look at where thoughts come from. It begins with a classic ACT exercise (Hayes, Strosahl, and Wilson 1999). We're going to tell you a fruit and ask you to remember it. The fruit is seedless watermelon. It's that simple. So if we ask you, "What is the fruit?" you'd say—make sure to say it out loud—"Seedless watermelon." It's important that you remember because, one day out of the blue, we're going to call one lucky person who bought this book and ask what the fruit is. That person could be you, and if you answer, "Seedless watermelon," we'll send you a large cash prize. Think about what you could do with that extra money. Again, you just need to answer one simple question. "What is the fruit?" Go ahead and repeat "seedless watermelon" three more times.

Okay, we actually don't have a cash prize waiting (sorry!), but if somehow we could call you next week and ask, "What is the fruit?" do you think you'd be able to say, "Seedless watermelon"? Probably. How about a couple of weeks from now or in a month or two? We managed to persuade you to repeat a phrase, and now you've got "seedless watermelon" rattling around in your head. And if we asked you to repeat these words daily for a week, you might have "seedless watermelon" up there until the day you die. Seems strange, no?

Let's explore a bit further. Read the phrases below and finish each:

Only the good die…

There's no place like…

Once bitten, twice…

We bet you said "young," "home," and "shy," right? But where did those thoughts come from? Like all thoughts, you came by them honestly at some point in your life. You weren't born with them. Throughout our lives, we're exposed to billions of words, from parents, peers, teachers, television, movies, newspapers, the Internet, and countless other sources, not to mention scores of images, videos, and life events, all leaving an echo in our memory. Each of these things is a potential "seedless watermelon."

Do you believe the thought *Only the good die young*? Probably not. It's easy to see that as an echo from the past. But what about thoughts that are more personal? Finish the following sentences with the first thing that pops into your head. It's important that you try not to edit, believe, or argue with whatever shows up. Simply notice the first thought your mind gives you and record it in your journal:

I'm overweight because...

My biggest problem is that I...

People find me to be...

I wish I were...

When you look at these thoughts, they probably seem less random than *There's no place like home*. Do they perhaps seem more true or real? Recognize that you also came by these thoughts honestly. Do you think you were born with a thought like *I'm weak*? Of course not. Can you recall or imagine when someone might have said this to you? Or maybe you deduced it by observing that other people seemed to handle things better than you or by comparing yourself to an imaged ideal.

The catch is that *I'm weak* is no different than *seedless watermelon*. You acquired both thoughts by simply living your life and being exposed to words. The difference is in how you relate to these thoughts. One seems silly and random, the other not so much. However, both are automatic thoughts, just echoes from your history that show up from time to time. What is the fruit again? Right. You're overweight because...? Of course.

Typically, people are unable to see thoughts as echoes of their history, which carries a danger. If *I'm weak* is real and true, then you have to change or make that thought go away before you can do important things in your life (the fix-me trap again). You have to fix *I'm weak.* After all, if you're literally too weak to follow a certain diet, there's no point in dieting until you're strong enough. So the thought needs to change before you can follow your diet. Unfortunately, thoughts don't seem to work that way.

Try to have the fruit *not* be "seedless watermelon." Go ahead. Forget that phrase and have the answer be something else entirely. That's pretty hard to do, isn't it? Now that "seedless watermelon" is up there, it's going to stay a while. There's no process we know of that allows "unlearning." Words and thoughts work by addition, not subtraction, so once you've got a thought in your head, you're likely to have that thought, or some variation on it, again in the future.

Now think about how brutal our society can be. Ridicule and judgment of overweight people is socially acceptable, showing up as fat jokes, stories about lack of willpower, shameful TV characters, magazines demonizing five-pound weight gains, and even friends and family members making disparaging comments. It's so bad, in fact, that kids start to show bias against overweight at age three (Cramer and Steinwert 1998). So if you're living in this world, you've been exposed to countless judgmental echoes, such as *I'm weak,* and they aren't going away. You've simply had too much exposure.

The other problem with trying to fix *I'm weak* is that efforts to do so validate that there is indeed something wrong with you that needs to be fixed. You're actually giving the thoughts more importance in your life, which is exactly the opposite of what you want. Thoughts are a part of you, something you experience. By treating them as if you need to fix them, you're back to the fix-me trap—a stance that what happens inside you isn't okay. It's like making yourself the enemy...of yourself! This isn't the self-compassionate approach we discussed in chapter 2.

Consider whether you can see *I'm weak* as just a thought— something you came by honestly, an echo of the past like *seedless watermelon.* If this is just repetitive chatter from your mind, the world's worst motivational speaker, you don't need to do anything about it. The thought *I'm weak* is natural and a part of you, but it's not the definition of you.

Seeing thoughts simply as thoughts can free you to behave in ways that are vital and meaningful to you, as opposed to focusing on trying to prove or disprove your thoughts. A key first step is noticing that all your thoughts are echoes. Some are helpful, some are unhelpful, and some are neither. Stepping back and seeing thoughts for what they are—just thoughts—can help you drop the struggle and empower healthy living.

The Diabolical Duo: Self-Sabotaging and Self-Evaluating Thoughts

If you're trying to lose weight, there are certain kinds of thoughts that can be particularly unhelpful. We call them the diabolical duo: self-sabotaging and self-evaluating thoughts. Self-sabotaging thoughts can be either positive (*I deserve this* or *I was good all week. Why not?*) or negative (*I don't deserve success* or *I've already blown it; what's another couple of cookies?*). Self-sabotaging thoughts encourage people to act in unhealthy ways. These echoes seem to pop up when we're vulnerable and encourage us to indulge or comfort ourselves. It shouldn't be surprising that we buy into these thoughts and do things that give us short-term pleasure or relief, even if it means sacrificing long-term goals.

The other half of the dynamic duo is self-evaluating thoughts—those that make judgments about your behavior, appearance, or character. Here are some examples: *I should have done better this week. There's something wrong with me. I'm disgusting. I'm probably going to gain the weight back.* These are particularly easy to get stuck on or struggle with because they seem to attack your self-worth. You may even hear your mind fighting for these thoughts right now: *But some of them are true!* Thank your mind, the world's worst motivational speaker, for chiming in.

EXERCISE: Recognizing the Diabolical Duo

Because buying into self-sabotaging and self-evaluating thoughts can easily get you off track, it's important to become more aware of them so you can recognize when they show up. Then you can change how you respond to them. Start a new section in your journal with the heading "My Self-Sabotaging Thoughts" and list as many self-sabotaging thoughts as you can think of. Go ahead and do it now.

***

Now think about your "greatest hits" of self-evaluating thoughts. Start a new section in your journal with the heading "My Self-Evaluating Thoughts" and list as many as you can think of. Go ahead and do it now.

***

How familiar were those thoughts to you? Do they seem old—kind of like a broken record your mind plays over and over again?

Keep an eye out for both kinds of thoughts, and when you notice them showing up, try labeling them as what they are: self-sabotaging or self-evaluating thoughts. You can say to yourself, *I'm noticing having a self-sabotaging thought right now.* Awareness is key. See the process as it happens.

Take a moment to consider whether these thoughts have been helpful to you in living your life the way you want to. Does regarding these thoughts as important or true help you live a vital, meaningful, healthy life? If the answer is no, maybe you don't need to buy into these thoughts when they show up. Maybe you can just make room for them without trying to control them or make them go away. Maybe you can simply notice them like you would a sudden gust of wind or a small animal running by—something noticeable, but of no consequence to you and the actions you ultimately choose to take.

EXTENDED PRACTICE EXERCISE: Watching Thoughts

The single best way to change your relationship to self-sabotaging and self-evaluating thoughts is to practice watching your thoughts. This is a classic ACT approach (Hayes, Strosahl, and Wilson 1999). Read through the entire exercise and then try doing it for five minutes.

Begin by briefly practicing mindfulness of your breath, as described in chapter 2.

After getting centered, close your eyes and imagine that you're seated about twenty rows back from a big stage. As you watch the stage, people with large signs enter from the left, walk all the way across the stage, and then exit to the right. On the signs are your thoughts, each on a sign of its own. Some go by slowly, others disappear quickly, and some may just hang out on the stage and circle around. Just let them go at their own pace, watching each as it passes through your line of sight. Visualize this scenario and watch your thoughts passing by on the stage for at least five minutes.

If the stage scenario isn't working for you, imagine each thought on a cloud floating by as you look up, or on a leaf flowing down a stream. If you find this hard to do for even just a few seconds, write your thoughts in your journal as they show up. Practice catching each one and writing it down, then do the visualization with the thoughts you recorded. As that becomes easier, you can skip the step of writing your thoughts and just imagine seeing them with your eyes closed.

You may have noticed that this can be hard to do. That's why it takes practice. Sometimes you might struggle with thoughts like *I'm not doing this right* or *I'm not having any thoughts*. Those are both thoughts, so see them on the signs moving across the stage as well.

Other times you might notice that you're no longer watching the stage. For example, you may notice the thought *This is weird* go by on a sign and then get lost in thoughts about what you have to do later, like *I need to buy bread*, and suddenly you're caught up in that thought. You're no longer watching the stage; you're on the stage. That's perfectly okay. The key is to simply notice that, then bring yourself back to the exercise and start watching your thoughts again. This is a key distinction to learn to make: noticing when you're watching your thoughts as opposed to when you're up on the stage caught up in a thought. You can always bring yourself back to watching. The goal isn't perfection; it's simply to train yourself to watch. This is the single most powerful way to change your relationship with your thoughts, so do this exercise frequently. We recommend at least five minutes of daily practice.

As you get more comfortable with watching your thoughts, see if you can direct your attention specifically to self-sabotaging and self-evaluating thoughts. Maybe those signs have different colors or appear in a different font. When you see one or the other, simply put it in a box with the appropriate label. When they are absent, just watch all of your other thoughts go by.

Getting Unstuck

The key with thoughts is to notice them and get unstuck from them. Thoughts can be like touching honey and then trying to wipe your hands off with a napkin. The stickiness remains. We can get stuck on all kinds of thoughts: self-sabotaging and self-evaluating thoughts, of course, but also painful memories, fears about the future, and stories about who we are and why we are the way we are. Your best recourse is to train yourself to see all of your thoughts the same: as simply thoughts. When you do that, you have the space to decide if a thought is helpful or not.

Thoughts can help you solve problems; they can also create them. Likewise, they can move you toward what you care about or further away. If a thought isn't helpful, let it be. Sidestep it, along with the need to respond to it, disprove it, or evaluate it as true or not. That's what we mean by getting unstuck: letting unhelpful thoughts hang around. It's okay. You don't need to fight or change them in order to take meaningful action in your life.

In addition to practicing watching your thoughts, various other techniques can help you get unstuck. Let's look at a few different kinds of thoughts and explore ways to get unstuck from them.

The Reason Brigade

We're culturally trained to give reasons for our behavior from when we're young ("I hit Johnny because I was angry"), to a bit older ("I can't get a date because nobody is attracted to me"), and all the way up to the present ("I didn't work out because I was too tired" or "I stopped dieting because I have no willpower"). In fact, countless times in your life you'll be asked, "Why did you do that?" You'd better have a socially acceptable answer, or people may look at you strangely. Yet from a scientific standpoint, why we do what we do is simply unknown. Seriously.

What did you do on the eighth day after your seventh birthday? How about the ninth day after your tenth birthday? You don't know? Of course you don't. The vast majority of each person's experiences are lost—inaccessible to memory and gone forever. However, let's assume for a moment that you remember everything that has ever happened to you. Even if you did, you still couldn't know the exact reasons you did or didn't do a certain something. For that to happen, your brain would have to be the most amazing computer ever, packed chock-full of accurate algorithms linked to known scientific principles of behavior (which don't exist).

Instead, we learn a sort of shorthand so we can peacefully and effectively coexist with other people. The stories we tell about why we do things, and don't do things, are for the benefit of society and not necessarily our own benefit. We can't go around saying, "I don't know," over and over. We need to hold people accountable for crimes and antisocial behavior if we are to function and live together. So we need markers to teach people what to do and what not to do.

For example, telling a child, "You hit your sister because you were angry. You can't hit your sister when you're angry," is a helpful learning tool. This will help the child realize that when he experiences a feeling he calls anger, he can't just hit people. That doesn't mean that anger causes hitting—that's absolutely not true—but that's part of the lesson such statements teach. Over time, we learn more and more "reasons" for why we do what we do, and we come to believe our own stories about our behavior. But problems arise when we believe all of the reasons our minds give us.

The more important question is this: Will buying into or believing a particular reason help you get closer to the life you want, or will it distance you? In other words, if you buy the reason *I can't work out because I'm too tired* or *I overeat because I'm addicted to sugar*, does that empower you to live a healthier life, or does it keep you stuck in old patterns? We understand that it may be confusing to think of reasons this way, as something other than preordained truths. Stick with us.

EXERCISE: Recognizing the Reason Brigade

Reasons can be like a well-trained military unit. They know their job, they're ready to be deployed, and your mind, the world's worst motivational speaker, uses them liberally to promote its agenda. Let's see how quickly your mind can call in the reason brigade. In your journal, write the heading "Reason Brigade." Then, without censoring or editing your thoughts, list all the reasons you can come up with for why you're overweight. You don't have to believe these reasons. Just list whatever comes to mind, and keep at it for at least five minutes.

***

How did that go? Our guess is that you came up with numerous reasons, and if we asked you to write longer, your mind could generate many more. When one unit is depleted, your mind probably calls in the next. Perhaps your mind leads out with the character brigade: *I'm weak, I don't have willpower,* and *I'm not strong enough to do this.* Then it follows with the history brigade: *I was teased a lot when I was younger, My mother forced me to eat everything on my plate,* and *My family loves food too much.* Close on its heels is the biology brigade: *I'm big boned, It's in my genes,* and *I'm addicted to sugar.* They just keep coming: the "the way it is" brigade (*I hate exercise, I love food too much,*

I'm Italian!); the logistics brigade (*I work too much, I don't have enough time*); and the "blaming others" brigade (*My partner doesn't support me, My kids take too much time, Nobody taught me how to be healthy*); and on and on.

We want to be very clear that we aren't arguing that any of these reasons are true or untrue, valid or invalid. Everyone has an understanding of how they came to be the way they are, and we aren't challenging your understanding of the way you came to be you. Rather, we just want you to look at a process: your mind's amazing ability to generate reasons.

Now we'll explore a bit further. Try to stick with this experience even if your mind fights back, as it probably will. Review the reasons you generated and see if you can group them in brigades in your journal. You can use the categories that we listed above or create your own. Number them, for example, "Brigade 1: History," and then list all the reasons that fit in that category. Then move to the next. Try to write comprehensive lists. Go ahead and do it now.

✱✱✱

How easy is it for your mind to generate reasons? We're betting it's really easy. You could probably go on endlessly. Now try this: Think about the reasons you have for losing weight—for better health, to improve your appearance, to feel better, to engage in desired activities, to improve intimacy, to be around for your grandchildren. In your journal, write the heading "Reasons for Losing Weight," then list all the best reasons you can think of. Go ahead and do it now.

✱✱✱

Does something seem fishy here? Your mind seems to be amazing at generating endless reasons. And you already seem to have powerful reasons to live more healthfully. If reasons actually caused behavior, then why isn't everyone at a healthy weight?

Here's a proposal: What if you loosened your attachment to reasons? Your mind will generate lots of them, some in favor of doing something, some against it. And then you get to decide whether a given reason is helpful in moving you toward what you want in your life. If not, you can simply let that reason be. Just watch it dispassionately, like you would a sign moving across the stage. Again, we aren't arguing that any given reason is true or false. That isn't the issue. The issue is whether buying into reasons is helpful.

Now notice if you have a strong attachment to any of those reasons. Can you hear your mind saying, *But this one is true; it's real!* Make a mental note of that. Those will be stickier thoughts, harder to notice simply as thoughts or echoes from your history. And as you notice attachment to any given reason, ask yourself whether buying into that reason has helped you move forward in your life. Has it helped you get close to the healthier lifestyle you really want? Has buying into that reason helped you find more vitality and meaning in life, or has it done the opposite? Maybe you can take a new stance in relation to the reasons your mind generates, allowing reasons to be present without having to behave consistently with them.

You, not your reasons, are in charge of choosing what to do with your behavior. For example, you can have the thought *I'm addicted to sugar* and still take steps to change your relationship to food. You don't have to make that thought go away or disprove it, and you also don't have to buy into that thought if doing so doesn't help you change your behavior in desired ways. To help you get disentangled from these kinds of thoughts, which we call sticky thoughts, choose one of them now. Write it in your journal, then complete the following sentences in your journal:

If I bought into that reason, I would...

If I chose to pursue what's important to me even though that reason was present, I would...

The Mind Rules

The play on words in "the mind rules" is intended here. It can feel like our minds rule us from time to time, often because our minds generate a lot of rules. Do any of these sound familiar?

- *I have to eat everything on my plate.*

- *I can't go to a party and not eat.*

- *I must feel more confident (in control, happier) in order to stick to healthy habits.*

- *I can't exercise in the morning (at night, when it's cold…).*

- *I can't work out in front of other people.*

Your mind, like everyone else's, probably generates a lot of rules. Sometimes rules are helpful (*Look both ways before crossing the street*). But like reasons, rules can also be unhelpful, and whether they are helpful can depend on the context. Rules are our minds saying, *No, I won't bend for you!* That rigidity can totally derail attempts to live more healthfully.

EXERCISE: Identifying Rules

Similar to the approach with reasons, we'll guide you in identifying the unhelpful rules your mind gives you. Here you'll generate a list of your mind's "greatest hits" of rules here so that you know what you're dealing with. Open your journal and write the heading "Mind Rules," then list as many rules that your mind gives you as you can think of, whether or not they are helpful. Go ahead and do it now, and write for about five minutes.

***

Now ask yourself whether having to follow these rules is helping you get closer to a vital, satisfying life. Is it moving you forward? If the answer is no, maybe you can recognize that your mind is great at generating rules, just as it is with reasons. Again, your mind thinks it's being helpful. Your job is to recognize which rules help you live the life you want to lead and then take action with your behavior. So take the list you just generated and write it out again, dividing the rules into two lists, "Helpful" and "Unhelpful," leaving some space between them. For each unhelpful rule, list one or two ways you could behave that are *inconsistent* with the rule and more consistent with a healthy lifestyle. Go ahead and do it now, and write for five to ten minutes.

***

Now pick one of those unhelpful rules and identify a situation where your mind is likely to remind you of that rule, giving you a chance to practice noticing the rule and acting inconsistently for the sake of a healthier lifestyle. For example, if the rule is *I must eat everything on my plate*, practice going to a restaurant, ordering a meal, and eating only half of it. If that sounds impossible, kindly thank your mind for that thought, and then choose to practice with your mind's constant interruptions. Similarly, if the rule is *I can't exercise in the morning*, go ahead and exercise in the morning, even just once, and notice how upset your mind gets in the process. The key is to let your mind do its thing—whining, complaining, and telling you that you can't—and to make room for all that chatter in the service of behaving in ways that matter to you. To remind yourself and make sure you follow through, write the activity you've chosen on an index card and place it somewhere you'll see it often. Go ahead and actually write the rule and the activity you'll do.

The "I Can't" Machine

Sometimes it seems as though when we're most vulnerable, our minds can turn into "I can't" machines. When we're tired, worn-out, stressed, or sad and need a little extra help staying on track with a healthy lifestyle, it seems our minds are especially prone to let us down with thoughts like *I just can't do it anymore, I can't do it today, I can't skip dessert at this party,* or *I can't prepare meals in advance.* You may even find yourself repeating these thoughts out loud: "Oh, I just can't... (fill in the blank)."

EXERCISE: Undermining the "I Can't" Machine

Try this game. Open your journal and write the heading "What My Mind Tells Me I Can't Do." Notice some that have come up recently, and some that are old and familiar and show up often. Go ahead and do it now.

***

Okay, before we continue, we want to emphasize that this exercise is just meant for illustrative purposes. Please don't take it too seriously!

Take a look at that list and ask yourself, if your closest loved one were held hostage right now and that person's life depended on you doing the things you listed, could you do them? For example, if a familiar "I can't" is *I can't exercise tonight because I'm too tired,* could you, in fact, work out if someone you cared about depended on it? Our guess is that in the vast majority of cases, your answer would be "Are you kidding? Heck yes, I could do it!" If there is anything on your list that you genuinely couldn't do, even under those circumstances, that's an actual "can't do." But the vast majority of times, things on the "I can't" list will fall into categories like "could do, but don't want to, don't feel like it," or "would be unpleasant."

Okay, now that we've got that straight, the next time you find yourself in an "I can't" situation," you can ask yourself whether it passes the hostage test. Often it won't.

Here's the catch, though: Your mind won't stop saying, *I can't*. It's an "I can't" machine. It's so well trained and so oriented toward short-term comfort, we know of no way to make it stop telling you *I can't* and start telling you *I can*. If you wait for that to happen, you might be waiting forever. So you have to learn how to change the way you relate to *I can't*. You can start by noticing when your mind goes into "I can't" mode. When that happens, imagine your mind as an "I can't" machine, remember that your mind is quite possibly the world's worst motivational speaker, and use any other exercise in this chapter that helps you get some distance from your thoughts, such as seeing them on signs.

The problem isn't your mind telling you, *I can't do this*; the problem is not seeing *I can't do this* as a thought. As with any other thought, you don't need to buy into it, behave consistently with it, or even change it. Step back from your thoughts, orient to what you care about both now and in the future, and make a healthy choice about how to behave, even when *I can't* is present.

You can practice this very simply. Pick up a pen and walk around the room repeating to yourself, *I can't walk around with this pen*. Do that for two minutes right now. The next time you work out, do the same thing; for example, tell yourself, *I can't go on this walk*, while you're walking. See if you can break up the connection between thoughts and actions so that later you can more easily get unstuck from sticky "I can't" thoughts.

The Mind Fights Back!

Your mind may be telling you, *But sometimes my thoughts are true!* You can notice that as a thought, but there's a broader issue here. To the degree you relate to your thoughts as true, you're at the whim of your mind. A thought like *I need to work harder* may be helpful to you in a given situation at a particular time; however, you can still notice it as a thought, something your mind provides. Relating to that thought as true and believing it whole-heartedly will keep you stuck in a cycle of behavior over the long term. That's why we often tell clients, "Don't believe your mind!" Believing your mind is what got you here in the first place.

You can notice your thoughts and choose to behave consistently with the helpful ones, but beware of the pull to validate them as true with a capital T. Once you do that, you also have to invalidate thoughts deemed false, at which point you're back to being stuck in your thoughts. You're also back to being stuck in a fix-me trap, where it's necessary to change or get rid of thoughts you don't like in order to then live the way you want. Don't get caught in that trap.

This approach even applies to the words on this page. Don't believe anything you read here. Belief is a part of the problem. Simply do what works for you in moving toward healthy living. If a thought is helpful, use it; if not, notice that, make room for the thought, and then move your feet where you want to go anyway. Do what matters to you whether your thoughts line up or not. Confused? Good! Confusion, pausing, taking perspective, and noticing are all helpful tools in getting unstuck from thoughts.

We recommend that you frequently ask yourself whether you're buying into unhelpful thoughts. Use this question as a way of connecting to the present moment—stepping back to watch the process of thinking, getting unstuck, and changing your relationship to your mind and the thoughts it offers up. This question can be a cue to apply everything you've learned in this chapter. We recommend that you keep a log of your unhelpful thoughts and any urges you have to act on them. Throughout your day, just check in with yourself and ask, *Am I buying into unhelpful thoughts?* If you have a smartphone, set an alarm to go off every couple of hours with this question popping up. You might be amazed at how helpful this brief reminder can be.

Going Further

This section contains two exercises designed to help you change your relationship with thoughts, getting unstuck from them and becoming more fully aware of the process of thinking, in the service of living more consistently with your values and goals.

EXTENDED PRACTICE EXERCISE: Observing the Lying Scale

Regularly weighing yourself can be very helpful for weight loss efforts. At the risk of stating the obvious, you need the information the scale provides to determine whether your calorie intake and energy output are in balance. In other words, if the number on the scale is going up, you need to make adjustments. Having the information is useful. However, you've probably had the experience of fearing that number. It's as if the number either completely validates everything you're doing or completely invalidates it. In reality, not much has changed. You simply got some information you can use. But the scale seems to be saying much more to you, like *You're disgusting, fat, horrible, and weak!* It's as if you step on the scale, and instead of a number, it just says "fat." We call that "the lying scale."

The scale can't tell you anything about your worth as a person, what you care about, or how well you're living your life. It just gives you a number. The rest is projected onto the experience by your friend the mind. And in addition to any insults your mind might throw at you, it may also say, *Oh, screw it! This is so worthless, I'm done with it!* That's a good time to thank your mind for being so invested in your well-being while also noticing what a terrible a motivational speaker it is.

One way to get the information you need without buying into all the nonsense is by simply stepping on the scale and noticing what shows up on the lying scale in addition to the numbers. Try weighing yourself every day for a week and keeping a log of the thoughts your mind offers. What does your mind say when you step on the scale? Visualize the thoughts popping up on an evil scale that's bent on ridiculing you and knocking you off track. This may help you see these messages as unhelpful content from your mind, rather than facts. In your journal, write the heading "The Lying Scale," and make a seven-day calendar beneath it. Each day, step on the scale and notice what the lying scale says to you. Write it down and note whether those thoughts are helpful or unhelpful.

EXTENDED PRACTICE EXERCISE: Busting Rules

This practice is an extension of the exercise "Identifying Rules," earlier in the chapter. Sometimes the only way to break the attachment to a rule is by deliberately breaking it. What's a rule that you feel you must follow? Maybe you think you can't wear mismatched socks or can't wear brown and black clothes together. Whatever it is, go ahead and do it and see if the results are catastrophic.

Also try this practice with food and choices related to your health and weight. For example, you might make a big plate of just veggies for dinner—lots of them, prepared healthfully and deliciously. Do you think you can't do this because it's not a real dinner? If so, do it and see what happens. Other examples would be having a healthy breakfast for dinner or going the gym and working out at a time when you think you absolutely can't.

Try busting some of these rules just to bust them. This doesn't have to be a regular practice, but do it enough to get you a little less stuck on rules in general. To remember this practice, choose the rules you'll deliberately break over the next week and write them on an index card. Keep the card with you or post it somewhere you'll see it often.

Summary

We live in a constant stream of thoughts. If we aren't aware of this, they can push us around. However, trying to control thoughts can be difficult, and research suggests that it may not be an effective way to deal with unwanted thoughts. Trying to change or fix thoughts leads to the fix-me trap, which further detracts from living a more vital, satisfying, healthy life. If, instead, you practice becoming more aware of thoughts and noticing them simply as thoughts, you can change your relationship to them and devote more focus to what you want to do with your behavior.

CHAPTER 4

Choosing Healthy Living Even When It's Hard

Dan had a stressful life. In addition to being a grade school teacher, he worked as an independent contractor servicing technology-based learning programs for schools. He also had a wife and three children at home. Dan was a self-described "stress ball." He felt like he was being pushed and pulled in every direction. Each day he wondered how he got through. It was like an out-of-control merry-go-round, and he couldn't hop off.

Dan's limited downtime was late at night, after all his work was done and the family settled down. His nightly wind-down routine included eating and watching TV. But once he started eating, he had difficulty stopping. Each day, a new round of busyness ensued, and he needed his nightly wind down again. Over time, this led to a lot of weight gain. He felt overwhelmed and didn't want to feel that way, but he didn't know what to do.

Dan was struggling with a problem many people face (your authors included): emotional eating. This is a clear example of the fix-me trap. We eat specifically for comfort or relief or to create more pleasant or tolerable feelings, if only for a short time. For example, if you find yourself eating something very tasty when you're sad, such as cookies or cake, you might be trying to change your emotional state with the immediate pleasure of food. Or perhaps you find yourself stopping for fast food on the way home after someone makes a critical comment at the gym or your boss gets on your case. You may not even be aware of how often this happens.

Emotional eating carries a key message at its core: *What I'm feeling is not okay, and I need to do something to make myself feel better.* It's completely understandable. Nobody wants to feel uncomfortable, whatever form that might take (stress, sadness, anxiety, boredom, and so on). And we all know that delicious (and often unhealthy) food is almost always available, usually with minimal effort and cost. No wonder people tend to turn to food when they feel emotionally unsettled.

Don't Worry, Be Happy!

For a long time, and indeed to this day, the cornerstone of therapy was to help people stop feeling sad, stressed, depressed, or anxious. The message was clear: these are abnormal or undesirable emotions, and the goal of life is to reduce or eliminate them, which presumably would lead to more happiness. However, psychologist Steven

Hayes made an interesting observation: it's really hard to feel good all the time.

Hayes and his colleagues conducted a number of studies on experiential avoidance. In plain language, experiential avoidance is doing something in an attempt to avoid, change, or control your feelings. It has also been called emotional avoidance. Hayes and his colleagues found that the more people engage in avoidance, the more problems they report having with all kinds of things. Typically, they were more depressed, more anxious, less productive at work, more troubled by physical pain symptoms, and so on, and generally had poorer quality of life (Hayes et al. 2004). This is why the fix-me trap is a trap: when we try to control what's going on inside, we can actually make things worse.

This led to a simple but profound revelation: What if emotional pain isn't the problem? What if the problem is attempts to avoid or escape from that pain? What if that's what really gets us stuck in life? ACT was born in part out of this discovery. And sure enough, in study after study ACT has helped people become less avoidant, and as they do so, they often become more effective at living in ways that are vital and satisfying (Hayes et al. 2006).

The ACT Approach

One of the key lessons of ACT can be boiled down to this simple statement: In general, we can all benefit from getting a little more comfortable with being uncomfortable. Does that sound silly? Let's examine it. When we try to avoid or change how we feel, we're essentially saying, *I can't bear to feel what I feel.* We can't (or don't want to) bear it presumably because it's uncomfortable in some way—a departure from a positive (or at least neutral or tolerable) emotional state. However, if you spend most of your limited and precious energy fighting how you feel, you won't have much left to apply to important things and what you desire in life.

You may wonder how you can shift your focus from managing how you feel to doing what's important to you. The solution is simple, if difficult: You can be *willing* to feel stuff. Experience whatever emotions show up, just as they are. That's it. This is what we mean by getting a little more comfortable with being uncomfortable. If you're willing to be uncomfortable, you might notice that you're feeling stressed and not have to focus your energy on making it go away, which frees you to spend your energy on what truly matters to you. Now you can be stressed and still take the time to exercise. Similarly, you might notice being sad and not require yourself to feel better before you can engage with friends or tackle a difficult work task.

While this is simple to say, of course it isn't so simple to do. First you need to dive deeper into how you relate to your feelings.

EXERCISE: Recognizing an Old Friend

This exercise will help you build acceptance of difficult feelings (Walser and Westrup 2007). Begin by thinking of a familiar, uncomfortable emotion—one that has reared its head countless times throughout your life, often when you least want it to. Maybe it's anxiety, shame, guilt, or sadness. Whatever it is for you, see if you can just get in touch with that emotion. In your journal, write the heading "My Old Friend," and beneath it, write your answers to the following questions.

What is the first experience you can remember of feeling this emotion, or something very similar? (Here's an example: "Shame: I first felt it as a little kid, but it wasn't about my body at the time. I remember being punished by my parents and feeling shameful.")

Now quickly calculate how old that emotion is. If you're fifty and can remember having that emotion when you were seven, it's about forty-three years old. How old is the emotion you listed?

Our guess is that the emotion goes all the way back to childhood. It's like an old, familiar companion—perhaps unwanted, but a companion nonetheless   that's been with you for longer than you care to remember. It's a fellow traveler. Many times as you've been walking your life path, it's been there with you. We ask you to refer to this emotion as "my old friend"—not to denote that you like it, but rather to acknowledge your intimacy with it. Calling it "my old friend" also has the benefit of changing how you relate to it, breaking up what's probably your typical dynamic: badly wanting to change or get rid of it. Like it or not, it's been with you for quite some time, and it will show up again in the future.

Despite society's messages to the contrary, constant happiness isn't normal. No amount of money, success, attractiveness, or anything else will produce it. Some of the most successful people are tortured inside. Some of the best looking people despise their bodies. Some of the richest lead empty lives. If you think of people you know well, you'll probably see that they struggle in at least some areas of life, and possibly many areas.

Think about this for a moment: every human being on this planet, every one, has an all-too-familiar unwanted or uncomfortable emotion—or two...or three...or more. They have painful feelings that are as old as they can remember and continue to arise from time to time.

Indeed, emotional pain is one of the few truly universal human experiences. It is, in fact, quite normal. There's virtually no way to avoid disappointment, heartache, and loss—unless you never try to do anything, never become intimate with others, and happen to have no family or friends. That isn't exactly a rich or meaningful life. And even if you could live in a protective cocoon, you'd still face random painful experiences. You may be thinking, *Well, that's pretty depressing.* We promise that we're going somewhere, so stick with us. Continue writing in your journal, working with the emotion you identified above and answering the following questions.

Where, when, and how has this emotion shown up in your life? (Here's an example: "I have shame about my body. It shows up when I step on a scale, look in the mirror, go the gym, attend social events, and receive subtle insults from coworkers, and during intimacy with my partner.")

What have you done in your life to try to escape or avoid this emotion, change it, or make it go away? (Here's an example: "I avoid the scale and the mirror. I only go the gym when I know few people will be there. I stopped dancing. I eat alone at work. I rarely have sex with my partner. When I feel shame, I eat soothing food, watch TV to zone out, and isolate from friends and family. Sometimes I preemptively make fun of myself just to get it out there.")

Take a good, long look at the list of things you've tried. Given all your efforts, have you succeeded in banishing that emotion permanently? Probably not. (If you have, you definitely need to write a book about how to do it!) We assume you're a reasonable, bright person. We assume that you've successfully solved many problems in your life. If you've made it this far, you're probably really good at solving problems. And yet here you are with an unwanted emotion that you can't get rid of permanently. You can't seem to fix this problem.

The question is, do your feelings really need fixing? Is treating yourself and your emotions as broken a compassionate way to live? Is it an effective way to pursue what's important to you? The choice is yours, but we suggest that treating yourself this way is a fix-me trap, and that it's likely to lead to more suffering, not less, and more interference with living your life, not less. In the next section, we'll look at why that's the case.

The Cost of Avoidance

Look back at what you wrote when you answered the questions in the previous exercise. Over the years, has this emotion become a bigger or smaller part of your life? When you consider that question, notice all the areas this emotion now affects. Using the example above, perhaps in an effort to manage shame about your body you started by wearing bigger clothes and avoiding dating, but now you notice that shame touches areas like how competent you feel at work, what tasks or challenges you take on, what you're willing to do for recreation (for example, you may choose not to dance or go to the beach), how you relate to family members, and your willingness to initiate or engage in sexual activity. So even if you tend to feel shame less often, shame might have grown in terms of its influence on what you do—and more importantly, what you don't do. If you're like most people, this emotion has become a bigger part of your life.

Avoidance can turn into a vicious cycle. For example, let's say someone insulted your body. You might be feeling a little sad, maybe angry, and perhaps a bit ashamed. The insult just happened to you; you didn't choose for it to happen, and now you have some emotional stuff showing up. This is an example of why emotional pain is unavoidable. You run into it simply in the course of living.

Once emotional stuff is present, you have a choice about how you'll respond to feeling uncomfortable. If you tend to try to avoid emotional pain, you might do something immediately to try to change or escape how you feel. You might drink alcohol, lash out at someone, zone out with TV, or simply isolate from others. People who struggle with food often choose to eat. It provides an immediate sense of pleasure that's even more reinforcing when unwanted feelings are present. It makes sense to turn to food when unwanted emotions are present. Food makes us feel good—thus the term "comfort food."

But what happens after you eat? You may feel guilt or shame, sometimes almost immediately. You might have self-judgments, such as *What's wrong with me!* or *I'm disgusting*. You may feel defeated and think, *I just can't do this. I give up.* So now you have some new stuff to deal with. But this stuff didn't just happen because of life; this stuff showed up because of how you chose to respond to the original stuff, the emotional pain of the insult. Avoidance itself created this new layer of unwanted emotional stuff. Herein lies the vicious cycle. Because what can you do to try to change or escape from all this new emotional stuff? Well, you can eat again, or perhaps do something else that doesn't support your health goals, like quit your diet, avoid the scale and the gym, and so on. The fix-me trap rears its ugly head. The more you try to manage your feelings, the more you create unwanted, unpleasant experiences, deepening the cycle.

We'd like to draw your attention to a couple of important things about this cycle. First, avoidance does tend to work, but only in the short term. When you eat cookies, cake, pizza, or potato chips, there *is* immediate pleasure—it does make you feel better. Remember that. We don't do these things by accident, we do them because they provide at least temporary comfort or relief. The problem is that this comfort is short-lived. And doing something unhealthy often unintentionally sets the stage for more emotionally painful experiences to show up later.

Second, as you engage in more avoidance behaviors, the cycle doesn't just continue; it also gets bigger. Imagine that your unwanted emotions are like a cute baby *Tyrannosaurus rex*. It's barely the size of your head. Its teeth can hardly bite through a doughnut. Baby *T. rex* comes by and snarls a little, and, concerned, you go ahead and feed him some meat to try to get him to leave you alone. As you feed him, he grows, and now he gnashes his teeth and roars. You have to find more and more meat as he grows and grows. You can't stop feeding him, because he gnashes and roars all the time now. It may seem like he can hurt you, but he never has; he's just so darn scary that you keep feeding him.

EXERCISE: Drawing Your Emotional *T. Rex*

We're going to ask you to get a little silly here. Imagine what your *T. rex* might look like and then draw it in your journal. Now put yourself in the picture (a stick figure is just fine, if you aren't artistically inclined), along with the pile of meat you have to keep throwing at the *T. rex*. Write the emotion (for example, "shame") on the *T. rex*, and write "avoidance" on the pile of meat. Then, on or alongside the pile, list some of the behaviors you do to avoid or escape from your emotions. Go ahead and make the drawing now. This illustration can serve as a metaphor for how you can get caught in the vicious cycle of avoidance.

***

We humans feed sadness, shame, guilt, anxiety, and other painful feelings by doing things to escape or avoid them. (That's feeding the hungry *T. rex* so he'll shut up and leave us alone.) As we do that, we strengthen the need to do it again in the future. Our emotions demand more avoidance of situations that might bring about discomfort. More things become off-limits. The reach of avoidance becomes greater the more we use it. And even as we get better and better at avoidance, painful emotions still find a way to show up, only now with added power.

Let the Good Times Roll

In addition to being a way to soothe difficult feelings, emotional eating can take another form: happy eating. Have you ever been having a great time with friends and then felt compelled to overeat? You may think, *This is so fun, you know what would make it even better? Pizza! Ice cream!* or *I'm having a good time. If I deprive myself of this food, I won't be having such a good time anymore.* That's the flip side of emotional eating: wanting to make good times feel even better. It's the sense that eating could enhance or maintain positive feelings. Just notice that there's avoidance in this too. The desire to feel better is a message that how good you feel now is not enough. The desire to avoid feelings of deprivation is a message that you can't bear to feel the discomfort of deprivation in this situation. In a way, it boils down to the thought *I can only enjoy this if I indulge all of my desires.* Keep this in mind as we proceed.

EXERCISE: Identifying Your Avoidance Strategies

Write a new heading in your journal: "Avoidance, from the Beginning." Then think as far back as possible and find your earliest memory of eating to influence how you felt, whether you were looking for the pleasure of eating or trying to escape an uncomfortable emotion. Write about your earliest memories of this for three to five minutes. Go ahead and do it now.

***

Now see if you can trace how the relationship between food and your feelings developed over time. See if you can identify when and how food became a way to influence how you felt or escape something uncomfortable. Write about that in your journal for three to five minutes.

***

Next, look back and find your earliest memory of a time when you didn't do something you really wanted to do because you were fearful, anxious, or worried about how others might perceive you. Write about that in your journal for three to five minutes.

***

Now see if you can trace your history of not doing potentially important, satisfying, or vital activities in order to protect yourself from fears, anxiety, or judgment, whether from yourself or others. These may be things you stopped doing, or they may be activities you decided not to try. Trace as many different areas as possible where this has shown up in your life over the years. For example, perhaps you're afraid of rejection, and you find that you refrained from going on dates, remained in a job you hated instead of applying for another one, and passed on attending certain social gatherings with people you weren't 100 percent comfortable with. List each area in your journal.

***

Now take a few minutes to draw a diagram in your journal. Write what you're trying to avoid at the center of a new page—for example, "avoid rejection." Then draw lines out to each area of life you notice this affecting. For example, if you notice that wanting to avoid shame keeps you from going to the gym, write the word "exercise," then draw a line from "shame" to "exercise." If you notice that avoiding shame keeps you from initiating sex with your partner or seeking intimacy with others, write "intimacy" and draw a line from shame to intimacy. Try to be as thorough as possible. Go ahead and do it now.

***

If you're like most people, your diagram probably reveals that avoidance of emotions has reverberations throughout your life. What if there were another way? Would you be willing to try something that goes against your natural instincts, something that forces you out of your comfort zone, if doing so meant you could change how you relate to your feelings?

Stepping Out of the Struggle

Letting go of an avoidance agenda can be liberating. What if you had woken up today and didn't have to manage your feelings? You're done with that. Whatever you feel, that's what you feel, knowing that you've had these emotions your whole life and understanding that you can live with them. After all, you already have for a long time. More importantly, what if you no longer had to choose what you were going to do based on how it might make you feel? What might you choose to do today? What are some things that have been off-limits for you?

This is your one and only life, your one chance to do what matters and what you care about, to connect with people and touch their lives, to seek knowledge, to grow, to laugh, to face challenges. You can do all of this, each and every day, by acting with willingness. That's the key to stepping out of struggle with emotions.

Willingness simply means receiving what's offered by life. When you take action in your life with willingness, you allow yourself to feel whatever you feel while doing what matters to you. You will experience emotions—sometimes pleasant, sometimes unpleasant, sometimes neutral. They will change—sometimes fading quickly and sometimes lingering.

Acting with willingness, which requires you to be a little more comfortable being uncomfortable, is a choice that will help you move forward in your life. And you get to make that choice thousands upon thousands of times. The goal is not to be perfectly willing at all times, but to act with willingness when you want to do something that's really important to you. You can act with willingness to adopt a healthier lifestyle and to pursue growth and vitality. To begin, simply make the choice to act with willingness more often than you do now. Let's try a small step in that direction.

EXTENDED PRACTICE EXERCISE: Welcoming Emotions as Old Friends

Read through this exercise in its entirety before doing it.

Begin by closing your eyes and practicing mindfulness of your breath for two to three minutes to get centered.

Next, bring to mind an emotion you tend to struggle with. See if you can act with willingness just for the duration of this exercise. During this exercise, it's okay for you to feel whatever you feel. Think of different situations in your life when this emotion has shown up. Picture a few of these situations, see yourself in them, then and there, and notice what's happening in these situations. Spend a few moments recalling these memories.

Next, see if you can locate where you feel this emotion in your body. Perhaps you feel it in your head or stomach, or as tension in your neck. Gently focus your attention on how this emotion feels and where you feel it. Notice how familiar it feels. You've experienced this emotion many times in your life, and you know it well. See if you can just allow it to be however it is for the duration of this exercise, without trying to change it or make it go away.

Start breathing deeply. On each inhalation, say out loud (or to yourself if you aren't in a private place), "Welcome" and then the emotion. So if it's shame, say, "Welcome, shame." And on each exhalation, say, "my old friend." Do this for two to three minutes: on the in breath, "Welcome, shame," and on the out breath, "my old friend."

By allowing yourself to simply feel what you feel, you're taking a step in the direction of willingness. You're saying, *Yes, I can stand with you*, to your emotions. You're saying, *I will do what matters despite how I feel*.

Come back to this practice often. With time, you're likely to find that you're getting a little more comfortable with being uncomfortable.

What You Can and Cannot Control

It can be hard to even see how or when you can choose to act with willingness. Imagine you're stuck in a room, and the walls are giant television screens all playing the same thing: your emotions. So, if you're scared, something scary is on the TV walls. If you're happy, something pleasant is on, and so on. Everywhere you look, your emotions are playing.

Now imagine that there's a remote control in front of you that's labeled "Emotion Control." It's big and confusing. It has a lot of buttons, and most of them seem to do nothing. In the past, when something has been on that you don't like and you felt uncomfortable, you'd try to change the channel or turn down the volume. When something fun was on, you'd try to keep it on that channel and turn up the volume. You've spent a lot of time focusing on that remote control. It seems like the thing to do. But doesn't your experience tell you that you ultimately can't control what's on the TV?

You've tried hitting buttons in every conceivable combination, and yet at best you've been only occasionally successful. When you were successful, you had to spend a lot of time pushing buttons to get there, sometimes hours or days. And just when you think you've figured out the right combination and sequence of buttons, suddenly it doesn't work anymore. Your emotions continue to come and go, seemingly at a whim, playing all over the walls.

At any time, you can choose to put down the remote—to drop the struggle. That would be acting with willingness.

When you do so, suddenly it won't matter as much what's playing on the TV and how loud it is. As long as you act with willingness, the TV is free to play whatever it plays. It could be a scary horror movie at maximum volume, and that might be extremely uncomfortable, but if you're acting with willingness, you no longer need to spend so much time with the remote, trying to control your emotions.

As you act with willingness and let the TV programs play, the first thing you're likely to notice is that the room seems a lot bigger—that there's more space than you thought. You have plenty of room to move around and to breathe.

More importantly, you're free to do whatever you want to do. Although you hadn't been aware of it, there are lots of other things to do in the room other than fixating on the TV screens. There are books to read, people to talk to, exercise equipment, games, and more. You still can't get away from the TV. It's going to be there playing what it plays, sometimes loud, sometimes quiet, but if you act with willingness you can choose to do other things. If, on the other hand, you're spending most of your energy trying to control the TV, you won't be able to do many other things. So, what will you do?

There are a lot of things we can't control in life and some we can. For example, you can't control the economy as a whole, but you can control how you spend the money you have. You can't control the weather, but you can control how you dress in relation to it. You can't control when people will send you e-mail, but you can control when you read it and how you respond.

The things we can control all have something in common: they are our behavior. The things we can't control usually involve other people or forces of nature. We typically don't question our ability to control the forces of nature. We've had a lot of experience in not being able to control them. Emotions are similar; they're mostly out of our control. But when it comes to our emotions, we tend to put up a fight—sometimes a lifelong fight, despite our experience of the futility of these efforts. We grab that emotion remote control and furiously hit its buttons, disengaging from our lives all the while.

Think of someone close to you who has struggled in life. Can you control that person's happiness? Of course not. Can that person control his or her happiness? If so, wouldn't that person simply choose to be happy all the time? Do you think there's something wrong with that person for not being happy? Probably not. But how about you? Do you think there's something wrong with you for not feeling happy (content, calm, together, confident, attractive, and so on)? Our guess is that, at times, you do think there's something wrong with you—or at least that's what your mind tells you.

You can't control whether a loved one is happy; however, you can control how you behave toward that person—for example, being kind, loving, supportive, or helpful. What if you have the same choice in regard to yourself? You can't control how you feel or when emotions arise, but you can control what you do when you experience difficult feelings. You can decide to act compassionately toward yourself, to act with purpose, and to do things that matter regardless of how you feel—if you put down the remote and choose to act with willingness.

Acting with Willingness

Willingness isn't a thing you possess. It isn't an attitude, and it definitely isn't a feeling. It isn't liking, condoning, or desiring negative emotions or bodily sensations. Willingness is an action, which is why we use the term "acting with willingness."

You're acting with willingness when you deliberately approach discomfort in the service of doing something important. If you exercise when you feel really tired, you're acting with willingness. If you go to the beach even though you feel terrified about how others might judge you, you're acting with willingness. If you make a healthy food choice despite powerful cravings shouting, *Give me that ice cream!* you're acting with willingness. If you initiate sex with your partner even though you notice powerful anxiety and fear of rejection, you're acting with willingness. These are acts of courage.

Sometimes it's hard to act with willingness because pain, fear, or the stress of the situation seems so overwhelming. It can be useful to slow things down and tune in to what's going on inside you.

Imagine you're scuba diving, looking around and seeing the different kinds of fish and other marine life. Suddenly, a giant fish, seemingly the size of a big whale, is coming at you. You can't tell what it is, but it looks huge and really scary. You can almost make out a giant mouth and beady eyes. As it heads toward, you think this might be the end, and you can't help but panic. The fish heads straight at you and then seemingly swims right through you. Only then do you notice that it's actually a giant school of fish, and the individual fish are small—each no more than three inches long. You see that there are thousands of fish, small, harmless ones, swimming over, under, around, and alongside you.

Intense and overpowering emotional experiences can be like a big school of fish. Together, they seem huge and scary—like they can do a lot of harm—but when you look at each individual fish and notice it for what it is, it feels less threatening.

EXERCISE: Seeing Emotions as a School of Fish

As you work your way through this exercise, pause after each paragraph to really get into the experience.

Begin by identifying a difficult emotion and a specific instance when you felt overwhelmed by that emotion. Get in touch with your memory of that situation and try to see it as it was happening then. Who was there? What did you see, hear, and smell? Take your time and bring as many details to your awareness as you can. Try to get in contact with the emotion and the situation in which it arose for at least a couple of minutes, until you notice that the emotion is present now.

Next, get in touch with your body and just notice how it's feeling. Think of your physical sensations as fish in the school. You might have several fish swirling around you. Do you feel a tightness in your chest, a pit in your stomach, or tension in your shoulders? How about your arms or legs? Is your mouth tight? Do you feel anything in your head? Mentally note each individual physical sensation.

Start with the first sensation, the first fish in the school. For example, if you feel tension in your shoulders, see whether you can notice it and simply drop any struggle you have with that experience. See if you can notice where that particular sensation begins and ends in your body. Trace it mentally. Then let go of struggling with it or trying to control it. Allow that tension to be, just as it is. Relax into the tension. We aren't asking you to like the experience, just to refrain from struggling with it.

After spending some time with the first sensation, move on to the next experience, the next fish. Maybe it's a tightness in your chest. See if you can just notice this second sensation. Put your attention on it, and as you do, see if you can drop any struggle you might be having with the sensation. Watch what your body does and notice where you feel what you feel. If other feelings or sensations begin to shove their way in, gently let them know that you'll get to them later. Simply notice the second sensation and allow it to be, watching it with curiosity. Continue to do this with other bodily sensations as you identify them. See if you can remain in contact with each for a short while, noticing that it's a single small fish.

Now see if you can notice any emotion you're feeling. Give it a name. Notice how it feels in your body, and as you do, see if you can allow it to be without struggling with it. Repeat the steps above with each emotion you can label. Notice each small fish and be present with it for a short time, simply allowing it to be.

Next, notice any thoughts you're having. Gently notice each one as it is, without struggle. See each thought as a small fish and gently pat it on the head. Note them as if you were making a catalog or inventory of thoughts. One by one, note each dispassionately and make room for it. Give yourself some time to do this. If you notice other experiences trying to push their way in, gently let them know that you'll get to them later.

Run through these steps with any remaining experiences: urges, memories, or additional sensations, feelings, or thoughts. Whatever is there, notice each experience individually. And as you do, see if you can let go of any struggle to try to change that experience. Try to do this for as long as you're able to notice new and different fish. Try to catalog the entire school of fish.

After finishing the exercise, open your journal and write a new heading: "My School of Fish." Then list as many individual fish as you can remember. Go ahead and do it now.

***

What did you notice as you pulled your experience apart? Did it feel different to deal with individual fish, rather than the whole school at once? Most people find it difficult to see the individual parts of an experience initially, but with practice you can break it down and make it more manageable. As you make room for all of the aspects of experience you naturally have, you can act with willingness and behave in ways that matter to you.

Building on a Foundation of Willingness

One of the things we like to point out to clients is that they already act with willingness, usually quite often, and probably every day. Think of the things you do that you don't necessarily want to do, or things that don't tend to make you feel good but that you do anyway because they matter in some way. Have you ever gone to work when you were really tired, upset, or worn-out? Of course you have. That's an act of willingness. You did it because doing your job matters in some way—maybe because you're truly committed to it, because it provides for your family, or because it gives you the freedom to do other things you enjoy, like travel.

Being a parent is definitely an ongoing act of willingness—as we know from personal experience! Kids require so much care, and that's a constant, even when you're tired or sad, when you feel like you're a bad parent, when you're scared, or when you feel helpless to comfort or influence them. Nurturing, supporting, and providing for your children, and ensuring their well-being even when doing so doesn't feel great or when they aren't giving you much in return—these are all acts of willingness.

For some people, every exercise session, no matter how long or short, requires acting with willingness. While exercising, you might find that you're making room for uncomfortable bodily sensations, the desire to just sit and rest, or maybe the stress of the day, as well as the nagging sense that you don't have the time to work out.

EXTENDED PRACTICE EXERCISE: Using the Willingness Pedometer

This exercise is designed to help you do two things: record all the ways you act with willingness right now, and increase the number of times you act with willingness. You're going to keep a willingness pedometer. Just like an actual pedometer, which tracks the number of steps you take in a given day, the willingness pedometer tracks the number of times you act with willingness. Think of these as willingness steps.

For one week, record each act of willingness, no matter how large or small. You can do this in your journal, a small notebook you carry with you, or your food diary if you keep one, or by any electronic means, such as on a smartphone. Each time you notice that you act with willingness, record it (for example, "Went to work feeling exhausted") and note the day and time.

Then, for the next week, continue to record your willingness steps and intentionally add one or two steps per day. Each day, identify one or two things you can do that you normally wouldn't have done. Do them and add those steps to your count. Pick actions that matter to you and that you know will make you uncomfortable in some way—situations where you'd usually be inclined to choose something easier or more comfortable. These don't have to be big steps (although it's great if they are!). For example, maybe instead of watching TV you could spend time preparing a healthy meal for the next day while noticing that you really want to just relax and zone out. Perhaps you'll choose to exercise in the morning even though you feel awful when you wake up. Maybe you'll take the time to call a family member or e-mail a friend even though you feel sad or stressed-out. In your journal, record any behavior changes you notice in yourself over the course of the second week.

Willingness and the Begging Dog

Willingness is like training a begging dog not to beg. If you put conditions on it, it doesn't really work. If you say you won't feed your dog people food *unless* he barks super loud or jumps up on the table, you're likely to get lots of jumping and barking.

If you put conditions on willingness, you're definitely not acting with willingness. It's more like you're sort of acting with willingness if everything goes well. Qualifying willingness by demanding that things go well or that you can't feel *too* bad isn't acting with willingness. When you act with willingness, your emotions are likely to push you beyond your comfort zone.

Acting with willingness is a bit like jumping (Hayes, Strosahl, and Wilson 1999). When you jump, both of your feet leave the ground and you put yourself in gravity's hands. This is true even of the smallest of small jumps.

Assuming you're physically able, put a piece of paper on the floor and then step off it, one foot at a time. Then try jumping off it with both feet at the same time. Although that's a very, very small jump, traveling such a short distance that it's almost impossible to measure, it is a jump nonetheless. You're taking your feet off the ground and letting gravity take over.

To act with willingness, you must commit to feeling what you feel as you take action. You can't always predict how you'll feel or how strong the feelings will be. You need to be open to whatever shows up.

To live in a way that's meaningful to you, you may need to do things that are quite a bit scarier than ignoring a begging dog. For example, acting with willingness might mean seeking physical intimacy while feeling disgusting, fearful, and shameful. That's a big leap, and it will be an act of courage.

Other jumps will be smaller, such as resisting cravings. Cravings are a lot like a begging dog in another way. If you relent and feed the dog, he'll want more the next time, just like the baby *T. rex*. The more you indulge a craving, the stronger it gets. Have you ever started having dessert after every meal? That's a really hard habit to break. Each time you have a craving and feed that craving, you're strengthening the association between cravings and eating, ensuring that the cravings will arise again.

Acting with willingness means riding out these cravings and their tantrums. When you notice a craving, try picturing it as a silly, big dog, whining and begging for a treat. Then try to act with willingness as you choose a healthier food or a behavior other than eating.

EXTENDED PRACTICE EXERCISE: Making Room for Cravings

Read through this exercise in its entirety before doing it. You can do this exercise with your eyes closed or open. You can also do it either by imagining foods that you crave or by having them present. We recommend starting with imagined foods. Practice that way for at least a week, then you can try having desired foods present.

Begin by practicing mindfulness of your breath for two to three minutes to get centered.

Shift your attention to a food that you're eating more often than you want to. Bring that food to mind. Imagine it in front of you—how it looks, smells, and tastes. Notice as many aspects of the food as possible. When you become aware of a craving to eat this food, move on to the next step; otherwise, just keep imagining the food and its many aspects until cravings show up.

See if you can describe one or two of those urges or cravings in detail. Just identify them and imagine throwing a spotlight on them. Become aware of how they manifest. What physical sensations are you experiencing in your body? In which parts of your body do you experience the craving? See if you can trace an outline of it with your mind's eye. What does the craving feel like in your body? What emotions are arising in relation to the craving? See if you can make a bit of room for those emotions and allow them to be there. Your enduring self can contain all of your experiences as they are.

Keep staying in contact with how you feel, and as you continue to get in touch with any cravings, see if you can drop any struggle with your cravings and just let them be. Like most people, you're probably accustomed to either fighting your cravings or feeding them. See if this time you can create a bit of room to make the choice to not act on any cravings now and instead act with willingness to feel those cravings, just staying with them and observing what's happening in your body. Imagine that you can expand around your cravings and make room for them inside of you without having to do anything about them.

Now imagine that your urge to eat is an ocean wave, and that you're a surfer, riding that wave of craving with your breath. Use your breath as your surfboard. Your job is to ride the wave from the beginning, staying with it through the peak of its intensity. Notice this wave with curiosity, and as you do so, notice whether your experience of the craving changes in any way. Have you ever just sat with a craving and looked at it, as opposed to reacting to it? Notice how you can simply stay present with this wave of craving, rather than immediately responding to it. Simply be present with the craving, without struggling or trying to make it go away, for another two to three minutes.

Willingness in a Nutshell: The Big Celebration Dinner

Let's explore willingness a bit more, this time using a classic ACT metaphor (Hayes, Strosahl, and Wilson 1999). Imagine you've planned a big celebration dinner. Your favorite restaurant is going to throw this dinner for you for free, with all of your favorite foods and beverages, in a private room. You and your guests can stay and celebrate as long as you want. There's just one catch: everyone you've ever met must be invited. Now, we're guessing there are at least a few people you would rather not see at the celebration. Try to identify a few of those people right now.

Despite that one drawback, you can't deny that it's a great deal, so you decide to go through with it. As the party begins, you realize that you have an amazing opportunity to connect with all of these people you care about, spending time laughing, catching up, and telling stories. But in the back of your mind, you're really hoping the unwanted guests don't show up. You look around, monitoring the doors to make sure those guests don't show. *They'll ruin this*, you think. *We could have such a good time without them.* As you keep an eye on the doors, you notice that you aren't as connected to the conversations you're having. Time is getting on, and you haven't talked to that many people.

Eventually, sure enough, one of those unwanted guests shows up. You think, *I can't have this person ruin the celebration, so I'm going to try to keep him out.* You go over and talk to this person at the door, trying to keep him out. You don't want him to ruin the event by making anyone uncomfortable, embarrassing you, or making you feel bad in some way. But it isn't easy to get him to leave, and you find yourself talking only to this one unwanted guest while the celebration goes on without you.

At long last he leaves, and you return to the party. But a few minutes later, he pops up at the back entrance. You didn't even know there was a back entrance! As the party goes on, you spend more and more time fending off more and more unwanted guests. In the process, you miss the celebration. You miss out on time with friends and family and the connections, stories, and laughs.

If you had let those guests in, they undoubtedly would have caused some kind of scene. They might have gotten a little too drunk, been loud and annoying, and spilled their drinks on people. They might have said something that made you feel embarrassed, angry, or sad. However, you would have been able to spend at least part of your time, if not most of it, how you wanted: talking to the people you care about and connecting despite the interruptions and distractions.

What if your life and weight loss efforts are like that celebration dinner? There's so much that you can do and experience if you don't fixate on unwanted guests. If you allow shame, self-doubt, and anxiety to go to the party, you can do any activity you care about: going out with friends, going to the beach, dancing, being intimate, freely expressing gratitude and love to others, and more. If you can allow cravings, stress, tiredness, sadness, and discomfort to attend the party, you'll find more freedom to choose healthier foods, eat smaller portions, and exercise more. All you need to do is act with willingness.

Going Further

Clients often ask us, "How can I be more willing?" It's a reasonable question. Unfortunately, we don't have a really good answer beyond the famous Nike slogan "Just do it!" Willingness is a behavior, and like any behavior, it takes practice. In the rest of this chapter, we provide several exercises for you to practice over time. Trust us, there's no way to be more willing (and therefore less avoidant) except to practice acting with willingness in uncomfortable situations. There's a difference between understanding willingness intellectually and acting with willingness, and action is what's crucial. What we care about is whether you're able to take positive action in your life in the face of barriers. So, practice, practice, practice!

EXTENDED PRACTICE EXERCISE: Carrying Your Emotion

Identify an emotion that you typically spend a lot of energy trying to change or avoid, such as shame, sadness, or anger—something where more willingness would create space for you to act more positively or effectively in your life. Write that emotion down on an index card. Keep the card in your pocket throughout the day as a physical metaphor for carrying that emotion with you. Twice a day, take the card out and notice any reactions you're having to that emotion. Write them on the back of the card, then put it back in your pocket and continue to carry it with you.

Check in periodically, asking yourself how willing you are to carry this with you as you pursue what's important to you throughout the day. Would you be willing to carry this emotion with you if it meant you could gain more control of your behavior? As you write more and more reactions on your card, just keep carrying it—keep living.

EXTENDED PRACTICE EXERCISE: Developing Awareness of Avoidance

The goal of this exercise is to see the behavioral choices you make and note how and when those choices are influenced by wanting to change or avoid an emotion. We recommend that you do this for one month, and then as needed thereafter. Create a simple tracking sheet, or just print out a blank monthly calendar. Each day, simply write the word "avoid" when you notice that you make a food choice motivated at least in part by wanting to change how you feel. So, if you're feeling stressed and think, *Eating pizza would make me feel so much better*, and then you actually eat pizza, write "avoid" for that day on the calendar. If you're feeling down and decide to eat ice cream because it will make you feel better or to pamper yourself, write "avoid."

As time goes by and your practice of willingness deepens, it may also be useful to write "willing" on days when you notice the pull to eat something purely for pleasure or comfort but instead choose a healthy food or choose not to eat. If you're keeping a food diary, you can simply add this to your calorie tracking.

EXTENDED PRACTICE EXERCISE: Seeking Out Your Cravings

Willingness to experience food cravings is a big part of changing your relationship to food. In the ACT approach, you're encouraged to create or approach situations where cravings are likely to occur; if you don't, it'll be hard to learn to do something different when cravings show up.

This exercise will help you do just that. We recommend that you do it often—at least once per week. It's best to approach it incrementally, starting small and working up to bigger challenges.

Since you're going to seek out cravings, start by trying to think of all the foods you tend to crave. In your journal, write the heading "Food Cravings," then list foods you often crave, starting with the most powerful cravings and ending with those that are less frequent and powerful. For one of us, the big three of pizza, hamburgers, and cookies would be at the top, with ice cream in the middle and burritos and potato chips closer to the bottom. (What, you think it's an accident we work in this area?) Use subheadings to categorize the cravings: "High-Craving Foods," "Medium-Craving Foods," and "Low-Craving Foods." Write as many cravings as you can in each category. Go ahead and do it now.

***

The next step is to identify situations where you encounter these foods or cravings for them. Write some of those situations beneath or alongside each category in your journal. Again, write as many as you can.

***

Now make a hierarchy of situations that you'll deliberately put yourself into for the purpose of exposing yourself to the craving while acting with willingness to choose a healthier option or refrain from eating. That probably sounds like torture, but here's the thing: you can't break patterns without…breaking patterns. The only way to do it is to do it. You have to get a little more comfortable being uncomfortable, and that requires being uncomfortable!

As you make your hierarchy, use these headings: "Somewhat Uncomfortable" (for example, going to a doughnut shop or bakery, purchasing a bottled water, and leaving); "Moderately Uncomfortable" (for example, going to lunch with coworkers, bringing a healthful meal, and eating it); "Very Uncomfortable" (for example, attending a banquet or social gathering with desired foods present); and "Most Uncomfortable" (for example, making cookies for other family members, leaving them out for four hours, and eating just one). Try to generate at least two situations in each category.

Over the course of several weeks (and beyond), deliberately enter these situations, and then choose to act with willingness. Start with the low-intensity situations and work your way up. Use all of the skills you've learned from this book. For example, when cravings show up, watch them mindfully, with awareness and curiosity. Notice something about them that you haven't noticed before: How do they really feel? Where are they located in your body? Do they change over time? Also notice any unhelpful thoughts your mind gives you. Really pay attention to how your mind ramps up its intensity, trying any little trick to convince you to indulge, perhaps assuring you that you'll make up for it later. Again, start with the easier items and work your way up.

Please note that the point isn't to refrain from eating desired foods completely. In fact, attempting to totally forbid yourself to eat desired foods can be harmful in the long run because they lead to chronic feelings of deprivation. The point is to practice acting with willingness and start having experiences in which you make a healthy choice. You can in fact make eating a choice. It's even okay to choose cookies sometimes. The key is that you do so as a genuine choice, not out of a compulsion to feed cravings or to avoid or indulge emotions or thoughts.

EXTENDED PRACTICE EXERCISE: Seeking Uncomfortable Feelings

This exercise uses the same concept as the preceding one, but in this case you'll work with experiences other than cravings: sadness, boredom, anxiety, stress, shame, and so on. In the same way, you'll seek out experiences for the purpose of breaking patterns related to emotional avoidance. Go through the same steps as above and generate a hierarchy of things you can do to deliberately expose yourself to discomfort in the service of doing something that's important to you or breaking a long-standing unhealthy pattern.

Become a pattern buster! Take steps to develop new patterns and reclaim your life from emotional avoidance. You can do it! Just be patient. Developing new patterns takes some time, along with a lot of practice in acting with willingness.

Summary

In this chapter we explored how patterns of avoidance can lead to increased suffering. When you try to run from how you feel, you're likely to find that you're less able to take important actions in your life. There's a good chance that you'll experience less vitality and satisfaction in life. Acting with willingness is the antidote. If you take courageous steps, whether big or small, to pursue what matters to you in life, even when doing so feels uncomfortable in some way and unwanted feelings are present, you can free yourself to be the healthy, loving person you truly want to be. The only way to get there is to keep taking steps toward what matters to you.

CHAPTER 5

Using Values to Build Healthy Habits

John thought life would be better if he could control his weight. It seemed the fit guys always got the better things in life. He figured that his best shot at being happier was to lose weight and have a great body. This became his mission. He was hyperfocused on counting calories and weighing himself. John became an expert at losing weight...and unfortunately also in gaining it back. He seemed to define himself by his weight, and expressed a lot of frustration with his struggles. During counseling, he often said, "I just want to see those damn numbers go down," as if bargaining with the scale.

John did what a lot of us end up doing. He became obsessed with the task of weight loss. If the numbers on the scale went up, he was upset, and if they went down, he was happy—at least for a little while. When he gained weight, he felt like that was evidence that something was wrong with him.

As discussed in chapter 1, you can't hate yourself thin, and as discussed in chapter 3, your mind is never going to be completely satisfied with you, no matter what you do. It can always imagine you looking better, doing more, having more success, money, love, and so on. Losing weight to fix what's going on inside is the fix-me trap in its most basic form, and it's not surprising that this ended in a yo-yo weight cycle for John.

The key thing about John's situation in regard to this chapter is that even when he lost weight, he never started doing things that would enrich his life, such as meeting new people, pursuing creative endeavors, or seeking a promotion. Instead, he just kept trying to lose more weight and get more fit. For John, the point of weight loss was to change how he felt about himself, and when that didn't work, food would, but only in the short term. Meanwhile he still had his life to live, and he wasn't doing that in a satisfying, vital way. There was an emptiness to it all.

The Importance of Why

Psychologist Kennon Sheldon was disturbed by repeated observations that people often set goals and then don't follow through with them. He also noticed that it was just as common for people to achieve their goals but feel no more satisfied with their life than they had been before. This suggests that, in general, people can be fairly unsuccessful in achieving goals and, interestingly, also fairly unsuccessful at picking goals that will enhance their life. Sheldon's work showed that perhaps the goals you choose, whether you achieve them, and whether they enhance your life are all related.

In a series of studies, Sheldon and his colleague Andrew Elliot asked participants to track the goals they set, whether they achieved them, and their psychological well-being, sometimes for as short a time as five days, and other times for months. They repeatedly found that goals that don't represent a person's deep interests and values are unlikely to elicit the sustained energy required to complete them, and that even when these goals are achieved, they're unlikely to provide the psychological benefits that might be expected (Sheldon and Elliot 1998, 1999). This dynamic is even more pronounced when goals are motivated by something negative, such as fear of failure.

The implication is clear: the *why* matters. Goals aren't helpful unless your motivation is personal and meaningful. Following a script of what you should be doing won't help you get the life you want. Trying to change your thoughts and feelings by accomplishing such goals will fall short. A more effective approach to living a vital, satisfying life is to discover what deeply and truly matters. This will empower your behavior.

The ACT Approach to Behavior Change

From an ACT perspective, identifying and cultivating personal, freely chosen values is the guiding light of all behavior change. If you don't have a deep understanding of what matters to you, you may find yourself in an endless and often empty process of setting goal after goal, with limited success in achieving them and little or no enhancement of your life.

So let's address the elephant in the room: Is weight loss important in itself, or is it only important in the context of living a life that matters to you? We'll tell you what we tell our clients: we don't care if you lose weight. We've written this entire book on how to help you live a healthier life, but we really don't care whether you lose weight. Are we crazy? Maybe. But before you decide, look at these epitaphs and tell us which one you'd rather have written on your tombstone:

"Here lies Pat, who finally lost those twenty pounds in the end."

"Here lies Pat, a caring friend and a loving parent."

We believe you'd choose the second epitaph. In the end, looking back on your life, your weight isn't nearly as important as how you lived your life, the relationships you had, how you connected with others, how you developed and grew intellectually and emotionally, and the joy you created in your life. We want you to live a life that matters to you. The question for you is how healthy living (and by extension, a healthy weight) fits into your life. If healthy living has a place in your life (and for most people it does), then we are 100 percent behind your success in losing weight.

Don't get us wrong. There is some inherent value in losing weight. Being overweight is associated with a number of physical health problems, in addition to social consequences. But the studies outlined above indicate the importance of your motivation for wanting to lose weight.

Most people say they want to lose weight for their health. But what does that mean? We want to help you clarify how being healthier will help you live the life you want to live. How does it relate to other important and vital things in your life? Will being healthy affect your relationships, your work, or your enjoyment of recreation? How will healthy habits help you grow into your true self?

We often hear clients say things like "I want to be confident," "I want to like myself," "I want to look great in a bathing suit," or "I want to feel more comfortable in my body." There's nothing wrong with wanting any of these things; the issue is that they are only means to an end. What would these things allow you to *do* in your life? Presumably, if you felt confident, you'd be living your life differently. The value is in living your life differently. So, what matters to you? What do you want to be doing?

We often ask clients, "What's at the bottom of that well?" because it could take many, many questions to find what's deeply important. Let's say you have the desire to be happy. Why do you want that? What would it get you? Perhaps you feel it would make you more confident. Okay, what's important about that? Maybe then you could buy nice clothes and like how you look. Okay, and what would that allow you to do in your life that matters to you? Perhaps then you'd be able to go out with your partner on a date or do more activities with your friends. At last, we got there! You value engaging your relationships fully.

Deciding to pursue health to appease a doctor or family member or to avoid criticism or ridicule from others won't help you maintain healthy habits in the long run. Think of it in terms of running away from something. Weight loss might keep a family member from nagging you, so you're trying to run away from the nagging and how it makes you feel (another form of the fix-me trap). It's the same with criticism, especially self-criticism. Running away is generally a short-term strategy. It may work for a while, but in the long term it doesn't.

On the other hand, being healthier might allow you to participate in activities with loved ones, have more energy to spend time with your kids, be around to see your grandchildren graduate, improve intimacy with your partner or spouse, do more things with friends, or perform at a higher level at work or in hobbies. You can think of these things as stuff you're moving toward. You want them, or more of them, in your life, and you're moving in that direction. If you can identify things you care about and truly value in the big picture, and keep them in focus, you're more likely to choose and achieve goals that take you toward those things. In other words, if you want to have more satisfaction and vitality in life, weight loss needs to be more about healthy living and the kinds of things that healthy living provides in your life, rather than solely about weight loss.

Healthy eating and exercise habits are merely an extension of a life well lived, and only you can decide how these healthy habits fit into a life that's driven by your values. In this chapter, we'll help you build patterns of healthy behavior that are consistent with your values and contribute to meaning and purpose in your daily life.

A New Way to Weigh Success: Valued Living

The first step toward joyful, healthy living is to identify your personal values. You can't build new, lasting patterns of behavior without connecting with what's deeply meaningful to you. Remember, this is about your whole life, not just your weight. If healthy habits don't fit into a broad set of values that give meaning to your life, then it will be difficult, if not impossible, to sustain new, healthful behaviors.

You might be thinking, *This seems like something we should have done earlier in the book.* This probably won't be the last time you have that thought! We do things a little differently, and there's a reason why we've taken some time to build up to this.

People tend to have a set of ideas about what they should be doing in life and what they should value and find important. This is heavily influenced by other people, such as parents, other family members, friends, and coworkers. Your mind, the world's worst motivational speaker, has taken these ideas and formed them into a big list of "shoulds." We all have our list.

We want to help you break through the "shoulds" and find your true self and what truly matters to you. Over the years, we've found that it's easier for people to identify core personal values after they have some practice relating differently to both thoughts (which you worked on in chapter 3) and feelings (the focus of chapter 4). It's too easy to fall into the fix-me trap with values too, choosing what's important mostly because your mind tells you that these things will make you feel better on a regular basis. The agenda of that approach is a life free of self-judgment and uncomfortable emotions, and experience has shown that it doesn't work.

EXERCISE: Identifying Your Values

With the previous discussion in mind, take a moment now to consider what matters most to you in important areas of life. In a moment, we'll ask you to write about what matters to you in four key areas of life, but first, some guidelines: As you write, try to note any intrusions from your mind telling you what you should care about. If it feels like a "should," it probably isn't something that truly matters to you. See if you can let that go and hone in on what you really care about. Also see if you can notice a pull to write things you think others might approve of. If you write something that would only matter if someone else knew you cared about it, that's probably not your own value. Try to focus on what truly matters to you, deep down inside. Remember that your journal is private: nobody will ever read what you write or pass judgment on it in any way. Finally, don't worry about having to write in a certain way; just let it flow.

Open your journal and write the heading "My Personal Values," then take some time to write freely about what matters to you in these four key areas of life, spending at least five minutes on each domain:

Relationships

Work or education

Personal interests (recreation, hobbies, your spiritual life, and so on)

Health

These four areas are important domains of life that many people care about. There are, of course, other areas of life you can choose to focus on, and we hope that you do, but in this book, we'll focus on these.

***

What was that like for you? Was it easy or hard? Did you notice anything that you weren't expecting? Were you able to let go of the "shoulds"? How about the pull to gain approval from others? Review what you wrote to make sure it reflects your own personal values.

EXERCISE: Writing Your Epitaph

This exercise is another ACT classic (Hayes, Strosahl, and Wilson 1999). Although it's somewhat morbid, it cuts to the core of what's missing when we focus on controlling our thoughts and feelings rather than living life. We're going to ask you to imagine that you've lived for many more years, happily and fully, and that your time has come to an end. This will happen to all of us. Our time is limited. raising a fundamental question that everyone faces: How do you want to spend your time on this earth? What do you wish to do with this precious gift of life that you've been given?

As you imagine being laid to rest, consider your epitaph. What would be a fulfilling epitaph on your tombstone? In a way, an epitaph is a measure of a life well lived. We think of this as the "epitaph test." Here are some examples that we feel do not pass the test:

Here Lies Julie...

She measured her life by how happy she felt.

She tried to make sure she never felt uncomfortable.

She chose the pleasure of eating over health.

She felt really self-confident.

She avoided everything that might make her feel self-conscious.

She spent all her energy fighting her weight.

Now, that list might include some items that you think qualify as a life well lived, such as feeling really self-confident. There's nothing wrong with feeling self-confident, and we certainly wouldn't discourage it. However, over the years we've found it to be a poor guide for behavior. It's simply too easy to turn "feeling self-confident" into "not feeling self-confident." The result is often some sort of internal pain and trying to run away from it (yes, another fix-me trap). When people are motivated to feel something positive all the time, this means really wanting to not feel the negative, flip side of that positive state, and that's a constraint. A well-lived life will include feeling self-confident and, by necessity, sometimes not feeling self-confident. After all, new challenges will bring doubts. A life free of self-doubt probably is a life free of challenge, and that's not a vital and satisfying way to live.

Now let's look at an example we feel does pass the epitaph test:

Here lies Donald...

He was kind and caring toward the people in his life.

He took on challenges.

He continued to pursue what was important to him when things became difficult.

He continued to seek opportunities to grow as a person.

He made a difference in the lives of his loved ones.

Can you see the difference? This second set is much more focused on behavior: what you do. That's something you can control. It's not focused on thoughts or feelings; those are things you can't control. To meet challenges and care for loved ones, you'll almost certainly have to experience unwanted thoughts and emotions along the way. It's part of the deal.

Now that you've seen some examples, open your journal and, continuing under the heading "My Personal Values," write an epitaph for yourself in each of the following domains:

Relationships

Work or education

Personal interests

Health

Make sure these statements represent a life well lived for you. Use what you wrote in the previous exercise for inspiration and ideas to inform your epitaph, and make sure what you come up with passes the epitaph test. Your statements should be focused on behavior, not what you think or feel. They should reflect how you want to be as a person, regardless of the opinions of others. Hopefully this will help you start cutting through the "shoulds" so you can identify core personal values that will sustain healthy behavior changes over time.

Finding Your Compass

A useful way to think about values is like directions on a compass (Hayes, Strosahl, and Wilson 1999). If you decide you want to move east, you can look at your compass and head in that direction. The moment you do that, you're heading east. You never actually *arrive* at east, but you can always check your compass to make sure you're heading east, and if you aren't, you can reorient and keep traveling east. Values statements are like directions. They're important for figuring out, in any given moment, what you want to be doing. After all, if you don't know where you're going, you won't get there.

An example of a values statement is "being loving and supportive." What are some things you can do to be loving and supportive? You could compliment your partner, help your kids with their homework, call your mother, attend events that are important to family members, help friends solve problems, and so on. If being loving is "moving east," all of those behaviors take you in that direction. Knowing your intended direction of travel can help you figure out how you might want to behave in any given moment. Notice, however, that you're never finished with being loving and supportive, just as you can never arrive at "east." Loving and supportive are chosen qualities of behavior, and you can be loving and supportive any moment of any day.

Values are different than goals. Goals can be very useful in helping you live in alignment with your values, but they aren't a replacement for those values. Getting a nice birthday present for your partner is a goal. But once you've gotten that present, then what? If you value being loving, you can always become aware of that value and figure out another thing to do that's consistent with being a loving partner.

This certainly applies to health. You can have a goal of losing sixty pounds, but why is that important to you?

What's that in the service of? If you value being healthy and active, that never ends, making it a great guide for behavior. In any given moment of any day you can choose to, for example, eat vegetables instead of a hamburger, or go for a walk instead of watching TV. When you do those things, you win! You're behaving consistently with your values in the moment. You don't have to wait until the pounds come off to live your values; you can live them right now, and in any moment whatsoever.

That's liberating. If you want to live a values-consistent life, you can choose to do so any day; there's no need to wait. And if you feel you've slipped, you can always begin again in any moment. If your values truly are freely chosen by you, reflecting qualities of behavior that you aspire to, then living in alignment with them is the most important thing—much more important than the numbers on the scale.

If, however, you only have the goal of losing weight, what happens if you achieve your goal? Do you stop trying to be healthy? And what if you don't reach your goal or the numbers on the scale don't go down for a week? Has your value of being healthy and active changed? Goals can be useful, but they're much more likely to be productive and achievable when they're guided by values. The key is knowing your personal values and using them to guide your behavior.

EXERCISE: Creating Your Values Statements

In this exercise, we'll help you develop some values statements. Imagine an ideal, what it would be like if you could live exactly how you want to live in the four areas of life you've been working with. What qualities would you choose for your behavior? Start a new section in your journal with the heading "Values Statements." We'll give you some examples here as well to help, but remember, your personal values are what's important here. Right now, take some time to write your own value statement for each of the four areas:

Relationships. *For example: Being a loving partner. Being a supportive and caring friend. Being a positive influence on my kids. Being a connected and engaged family member.*

Work or education. *For example: Continuing to learn and grow throughout life. Being a reliable, caring worker. Being a supportive coworker. Contributing to the education and mentorship of others.*

Personal interests. *For example: Behaving in ways that support spiritual growth. Being kind and charitable. Being playful. Taking on challenges.*

Health. *For example: Being active and engaged. Being mindful of how my behavior affects my health. Providing the nourishment and self-care that fosters long-term health.*

As mentioned, values statements should help you decide how you want to behave in a given situation. They should also be action oriented. That's why our examples often start with "being." Read through your statements, and if you can't identify ten ways to behave consistently with any of them—ten actual behaviors you could do—go back and try to rewrite the statement so it will provide that kind of guidance.

Here's another test of a values statement: Think of a time when it would be hard to behave in alignment with a particular values statement—perhaps a time when you're upset with your partner or a family member. Then look at your values statement in regard to relationships and imagine what you could do that would be consistent with your statement even though you're upset. For example, you may be upset that your partner isn't helping out enough around the house. Yelling at your partner wouldn't be consistent with that value. However, calmly expressing your needs while also noting how appreciative you are of other things your partner does is fairly consistent with being loving and supportive. In hard situations, values statements should point you toward more compassionate and effective behavior.

Take one last look through your values statements and make sure they fit the criteria above. Ultimately, they should be useful to you. If they're not, keep working on them.

EXTENDED PRACTICE EXERCISE: Aiming for Valued Living

This exercise uses a bull's-eye diagram (adapted with permission from Dahl and Lundgren 2006) to help you track how consistent your behaviors are with your values. Each quadrant represents one of the areas of life you've been working with in this chapter. The idea is to use the diagram to create more balance among these four areas, which can help foster a healthy, vital, satisfying life.

Here's the basic diagram. We recommend that you fill it out once a week, so please photocopy it so you can use it repeatedly.

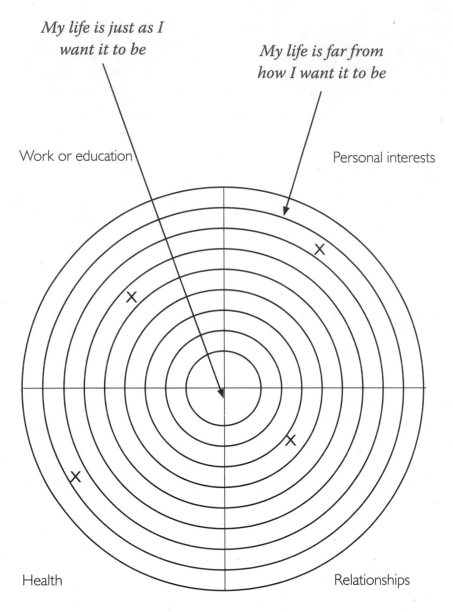

My life is just as I want it to be

My life is far from how I want it to be

Work or education

Personal interests

Health

Relationships

To use the diagram, first review the values statements you've written. Write your values statement for each domain next to the relevant quadrant. Then put an X in each quadrant to indicate how consistently you lived with each values statement over the past week. Think of a bull's-eye (the innermost circle) as living totally and completely in alignment with that value. If you feel that your behavior is farther away from your ideal, then mark an X more toward the outside of the target. Keep in mind that an X in the bull's-eye at the center of the diagram doesn't mean you're always feeling great and thinking positive thoughts, or that you're perfectly successful in every endeavor; rather, it means you're behaving exactly how you want to behave, regardless of how things are going. Here's an example based on John's story, from the beginning of this chapter:

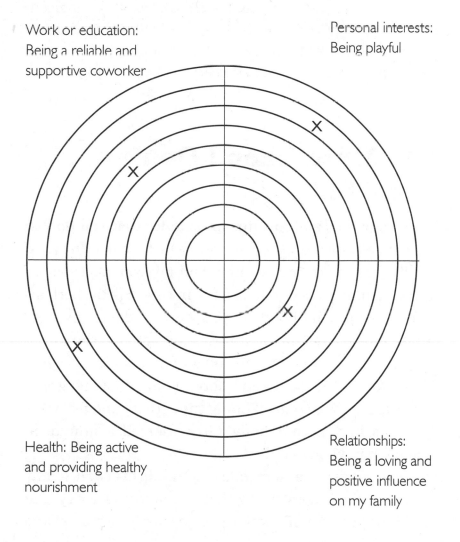

Work or education: Being a reliable and supportive coworker

Personal interests: Being playful

Health: Being active and providing healthy nourishment

Relationships: Being a loving and positive influence on my family

This diagram reveals that John's doing very well in relationships, but less so in the domains of work, health, and personal interests. So John might use this diagram to orient himself toward his values before and during work, and also when he eats meals and at night. Don't try to get every X to the center immediately; that's asking too much of yourself. It can be helpful to pick one area to focus on for a week, then check back at the end of the week to see whether you're living more consistently with your values in that area.

Now it's your turn. Go ahead and mark four Xs on the dartboard based on how closely you think your behaviors have aligned with your values over the past week. Continue to use the bull's-eye diagram, filling it out every week to check in with your progress.

"If I Must, Then I Don't Want To!"

Close your eyes and imagine an activity that you do just for yourself, for no other reason than that it brings joy, vitality, or growth to your life. And no, you can't choose eating! You may need to look back in time a little, perhaps even to your childhood, if you haven't done anything purely for yourself for a while. This activity should be something that's for you and you alone—something you'd do even if no one could know about it and it had no grand purpose. Imagine yourself doing the activity and feel what that feels like in your body. Give yourself a minute to imagine it in vivid detail.

Now imagine that someone is standing over you, loudly and aggressively demanding that you do this activity. You must now perform this activity to appease this person and others who are watching. Notice how that feels. Give yourself a minute to really tune in to that.

Did you feel a difference? Although you're imagining the same activity, it probably felt very different in the two scenarios. Your motivation is quite different in the two situations. First you were doing something meaningful to you, then you were doing something out of a sense of obligation or because you felt forced to do it.

You've probably experienced this many times in life. Maybe in school you picked up a book that you thought looked fun and interesting, but then you found out you'd be tested on it and everything changed. It was the same book, but your motivation changed from genuine interest to task-oriented performance anxiety. Suddenly it wasn't a choice to read that wonderful book, you had to...or else. This is exactly what happens with healthy activities, except with these, we often are the ones standing over ourselves and yelling, *You must do this!*

We human beings are meant to dance and jump and run and revel. Watch children at play, and you can see the joy they take in simply being active. Unfortunately, people tend to contaminate these joyful activities with the shackles of demands, expectations for performance, and "shoulds." We sentence ourselves to soul-sucking diets and exercise regimens because we "have to," because our bodies are "disgusting," or because of the thought *I can't feel this way anymore.* You might as well hire someone to stand over you and yell, "Perform, prisoner!" Obviously, this context isn't conducive to experiencing the joy of healthy living.

Perhaps you recognize that person yelling at you internally. Maybe that person is your mind, the world's worst motivational speaker; or perhaps it's an echo of your parents or partner. You might need to practice some of the new skills you've learned to help you find a more vital path along the way (for example, noticing your thoughts simply as thoughts).

Turning "I Must" into "I Choose"

You've undoubtedly heard the phrase "can't see the forest for the trees." That saying has a lot of relevance for weight loss. When people are fixated on rigid rules, it's no wonder that they don't find much joy in healthy living. They're so focused on the trees right in front of them that they fail to see the beautiful forest, rich with foliage and wildlife.

One of the most wonderful things about values is how they help expand your time horizon, helping you see the forest, so to speak. Valued living is about doing what's best for you in the long run, rather than what feels good in the moment. Connecting to your values during any activity will help you shift your focus from any discomfort and resistance you're feeling in the moment (the tree right in front of you) to how the activity fits into the vital and satisfying life you've chosen (the majestic forest).

Imagine that you're running on a treadmill for thirty minutes, and all you think about is how you have to do it because it's a part of your weight loss plan. That's it. You must lose weight, and to do so you must work out. Now imagine working out for thirty minutes while in touch with what exercise offers or holds. Perhaps you know that exercising regularly helps you sleep better at night, which allows you to function better both at work and at home, supporting your value of being an active and engaged family member, friend, and coworker. Furthermore, consistent exercise gives you more energy for running in a 5K fund-raiser for cancer research, and for playing with your children or grandchildren—not to mention that it would be nice to be around (and lucid and mobile!) to see your kids or grandkids graduate from college.

If you're exercising in service of all of those wonderful things, that's a different and much richer story than "I must lose another pound." Remember, you get to choose. It's your life, so do what matters to you.

Think of all the things you tell yourself you "have to do." If some of those things don't fit with your values, maybe you can let some of them go. Honestly, if you find absolutely no personal meaning in a given activity, it's okay to let go of it. However, give yourself a chance to find any meaning first.

We bet that many healthy behaviors do hold meaning for you, and that if you were able to see the forest (connect to your values), it would transform the experience of doing these activities, making them richer and more vital. You can turn "I must" into "I choose" if you orient to what's important to you within those actions. Here's an example of a day that includes many potential instances of "I must" that can be turned into "I choose" by adding the context of values.

Life areas	"I must"	I choose (What's the value?)
Health and relationships	*Making my family breakfast*	*Acting with love. Helping them get a healthy start to the day. Being a loving and supportive parent.*
Work	*Completing reports*	*Providing for my family. Supporting my coworkers. Building my skill set.*
Health	*Eating a healthy lunch*	*Providing my body with energy and nutrition to foster a long, healthy life.*
Relationships	*Picking up my kids*	*Being engaged with my children. Listening and interacting with them in the time I have to spend with them.*
Health and personal interests	*Walking for exercise*	*Being active and engaged. Taking care of my body.*

EXTENDED PRACTICE EXERCISE: Choosing to Do Things That Matter

Start a new section in your journal with the title "I Choose." Now make a list of things you do that are consistent with your values but often feel like obligations, or "must dos." As in the preceding table, choose activities that you often find difficult to do, that you try to whip yourself into doing, or that you do solely out of obligation—or simply things you do solely in the service of the narrow task of weight loss. Then look at your bull's-eye diagram and the values statements you've generated and use them as your compass. Identify and connect to why these activities are important and vital for you. Then write the values within each activity—the "I choose" qualities. Pick at least one behavior from each of the four domains and write the values behind it. Go ahead and do it now.

***

It can be easier to engage in healthy behaviors if you consult your compass and remind yourself why you've chosen these behaviors. And, equally importantly, remind yourself that you're choosing to do these things. Try doing this for a week and then continue for to do it as long as you find it useful.

Staying Persistent

Once you start moving in the direction you want, toward a healthy, vital life, you'll need to stick with those behaviors long enough to get your reward. It's like running; many people say it takes one to two miles before they reach a sense of flow or joy in running.

Much of the reward of exercise lies in how it impacts your day-to-day functioning by developing your strength, giving you more energy, helping you sleep better, and so on. This is very different from the immediate reward of eating chocolate. You don't have to wait for that at all! The things that are most meaningful and valuable in life often require time and patience.

How persistent are you in the face of difficulties? When you think of how you want to behave (not how much money you have or how successful you are in work and relationships, but just how you want to be behaving), what stops you from living just like that, fully and vitally? Typically, the barriers are the kinds of things dealt with in chapters 3 and 4: unwanted thoughts, feelings, and bodily sensations, such as anxiety, fear of failure, thoughts of not being good enough, strong urges, or fatigue.

Persistence means continuing in the face of these barriers. It too is a choice—a choice to keep going when your mind starts beating you up or telling you to quit. It's a choice to keep going when you experience powerful emotions that you wish to escape or cravings that beg to be indulged. The reason to persist is that it furthers your values. Values-consistent behavior is the key to a vital life worth living, and to becoming what you aspire to be. Persistence is an act of courage.

EXTENDED PRACTICE EXERCISE: Being Still

This exercise will help you train your persistence and practice sitting with discomfort. Read through the exercise in its entirety before doing it.

Begin by sitting in a quiet place and paying attention to the fact that your body is actively sensing the environment. Then practice mindfulness of your breath for two minutes. If you become distracted by your thoughts, just take a moment to notice where your thoughts took you, and then, without judgment, let go of those thoughts and return your attention to your breathing. Do this throughout the exercise anytime you find your mind wandering.

Turn your full attention to your body. Starting with your toes, scan up your body slowly, all the way to the top of your head. Take a couple of minutes to do this, briefly pausing each time you notice a new sensation. As you pay attention to your body, practice remaining perfectly still except for the rise and fall of your chest and abdomen as you breathe. You may notice that you have an itch, a desire to move, or some discomfort, but your task at this time is to simply notice those desires and sensations without trying to make them different. Stay still… Simply watch as your mind, body, and emotions ask you to do something, and also notice that you can remain perfectly still despite these requests.

Continue to remain still as you notice the different sensations in your body, becoming aware that you don't need to react to sensations; you can simply observe them. Just watch them come and go. You don't need to feel a certain way or think certain thoughts; you only need to remain still. Continue to do this for about ten minutes.

We recommend practicing this exercise regularly over the coming weeks and months. It will help you develop persistence in the face of discomfort.

Showing Yourself Gratitude

As you begin to establish new, healthy habits, it's important to extend gratitude to yourself for your efforts. As discussed, the human mind has a tendency to be highly critical. Even if you complete twenty tasks today, your mind might reprimand you for not doing forty. Practice showing gratitude to yourself for your accomplishments and forgiving yourself when things haven't gone so well.

EXERCISE: Writing a Letter of Gratitude

An easy way to foster vitality is to write a letter of gratitude to yourself. It's more powerful than merely taking a few moments to think about things. When you write to yourself as you were earlier that day, you actually introduce another perspective that's more healthy and loving.

Take a moment now to identify five values-consistent behaviors you've done today. They can be small (eating a healthy breakfast or helping a coworker with a task at work) or bigger (taking a two-hour walk, or supporting a loved one through an emotionally difficult experience). Then briefly write from the perspective of yourself, here and now, thanking you, there and then, for doing those things in those earlier moments. Also express gratitude to yourself for everything you do in the face of difficulty. Go ahead and write the letter now.

***

What did you notice as you wrote the letter? Did your mind try to convince you that you don't deserve the gratitude or that what you did wasn't important enough? If so, that's okay. When that happens, you can thank your mind for intruding and continue offering gratitude to yourself. Did it feel uncomfortable to express gratefulness to yourself? That's also okay; you're probably not used to doing this. Extending gratitude to yourself is an act of self-compassion, and it takes practice. See if you can practice little acts of gratitude toward yourself throughout the week.

Eating Is Not Gratitude

We made this point earlier, but it bears repeating: Eating salty, fatty, sugary foods isn't gratitude, and it isn't self-compassion. It's exactly the opposite. One of the most common pitfalls among our clients is revealed by statements like "I decided I wasn't going to deny myself" or "It was such a bad day that I had to treat myself." Of course, there's nothing wrong with having less-than-healthful foods from time to time, particularly if you plan for them and fit them into your lifestyle. But eating high-calorie foods in the name of self-compassion is just avoidance disguised as gratitude. It's a classic example of the fix-me trap. Eating to soothe yourself or make a craving go away, as opposed to eating to nourish your body, is an act that says, *I don't like how I feel. It's not okay to feel this way, and I must change it.* Don't confuse eating with genuine gratitude and restorative acts of kindness, no matter what your mind tells you! Restorative acts of kindness include taking a scenic walk, engaging with friends and loved ones, spending some quiet alone time doing a recreational activity such as reading, or doing any activity that's enjoyable to you and doesn't contribute to poor physical health or serve the function of helping you avoid how you feel.

Beyond Weight Loss: Pressing the Play Button on Life

Building healthy habits in regard to relationships, work, personal interests, and growth are just as important as weight loss, if not more important, in the pursuit of a more vital life. Again, if you're just focused on the narrow task of weight loss, you're likely to be missing the big picture. One of the best ways to improve your overall health is to live your values by focusing on things that matter other than just controlling your weight.

It's easy to fall into the trap of working on your weight so that *then* you can have the life you want. Again, this is a fix-me trap. You get to live your ideal life only when you've "fixed" whatever you perceive is wrong with your body, which presumably will lead to more positive thoughts and feelings about yourself. It isn't surprising that people fall into this trap. After all, it's the familiar refrain of diet programs: "Look better, feel better, and then you can have a great life!" We sincerely hope that this now sounds like poppycock to you.

Even if you don't buy into the fix-me agenda anymore, you may have fallen into that trap before reading this book. There's a good chance you pressed the pause button on life in at least some areas. We want to turn that script around. If you haven't started already, it's time to push the play button on life again. Right now, today, you can decide to do the things that you care about, to live consistently with your values, to seek what's important to you, regardless of feelings of shame or embarrassment, self-judgments about your weight and how you look, or fear of what others might think of you. You can let go of the struggle to win the war with how you think and feel and instead focus on pursuing what matters to you. There's nothing stopping you. It's a choice—and it's a choice that you get to make again and again. Each moment is a new opportunity to make that choice, no matter what came before.

EXTENDED PRACTICE EXERCISE: Pressing the Play Button

Take a moment to review the values statements you've written in your journal, then reflect on your life in recent months or years and identify at least three ways you've pushed the pause button on life. These would be things that you enjoy or could enjoy and that matter to you, but that you've put off or stopped doing because of your weight or because of unwanted thoughts or feelings, such as self-judgment or anxiety, or fear of such thoughts and feelings. Typical examples include dancing, making new friends, going to the beach, going out with coworkers, swimming, intimacy, pursuing new interests, volunteering, connecting with certain friends or family members, taking a class, starting a new hobby, or a spiritual practice. Of course, we're all unique, and the activities you haven't pursued may be completely different. In your journal, write the heading "Pushing the Pause Button on Life," then list three ways in which you've done this.

Next, take a few moments to identify three to five things you can start doing right now that would be consistent with your values statements and help you get closer to the bull's-eye in your life. They don't have to be grand endeavors, though we do encourage you to be really bold! Most important is that they be steps in the direction of a more vital life, and that they get you to take action in areas where you've pushed the pause button on life. Write the heading "Pushing the Play Button on Life" in your journal, and list these new actions beneath it.

We ask that you commit to doing these things—to pressing the play button on life—over the next week. And don't be content with these three actions. As time passes, continue to identify ways—both large and small—that you can live the life you want to live *right now*. Then add them to your list and commit to doing them.

At the end of each week, when you fill out a new bull's-eye diagram, also check off whether you did these new activities. If you have, be sure to come up with a few new ones for the next week. If not, try to identify what got in the way. Are there thoughts that you can practice relating to in a different way, as outlined in chapter 3? Or perhaps you notice that a lack of willingness is getting in the way, in which case you might want to revisit chapter 4. Your mind will probably say things like *I'm too busy to do that*, and those thoughts may even be valid in a sense. But if you look closely, thoughts and feelings, or the desire to avoid them, are probably playing a role. Even buying into the thought *I'm too busy* is a part of the equation. Make a special effort to look for thoughts and feelings, or desires to avoid them, that may be showing up as a barrier. Try to come from the standpoint that this is definitely happening, and that you're a detective who's trying to find out how thoughts and feelings are getting in the way. The tendency to avoid painful thoughts and feelings is very strong, and your mind will create stories to help you avoid them, so it's a good idea to be on the lookout for this.

EXERCISE: Finding Meaning in Pain

We've focused on you and your behavior throughout this chapter. There are some other important pieces of this puzzle: everyone and everything else! We can't honestly say, "Just pursue what matters and everything will be great!" That's not the way the world works. You can do a lot of excellent work and still not get a promotion. You can open yourself up and be betrayed by your partner. You can be supportive of a family member and receive criticism in return. Life involves pain, without question.

Take a moment now to remember a time when someone close to you really hurt you. What happened? Why did it hurt so much? Start a new section in your journal with the title "Remembering Pain," and write for about five minutes about what happened and how it affected what you did and how you lived afterward. Go ahead and do it now.

***

We have a saying in ACT: In your pain you find your values, and in your values you find your pain. In other words, if you didn't care, it wouldn't hurt. If you love your partner, your partner can hurt you by cheating on you, ridiculing you, or not being supportive. It hurts precisely because you care. You probably value engaging in honest, supportive, mutually satisfying relationships. When you care, there's the potential for pain. To not have pain, you'd have to not care about the relationship.

The flip side, of course, is that if you didn't care about relationships, you might not experience that pain, but you also couldn't experience any of the wonderful aspects of connecting with others. To experience love, joy, and support, you must be open to it and care about it. That makes you vulnerable to pain.

Your mind wants to protect you from pain. Let's say your partner cheated on you. Your mind might come in and say, *That's it. I'm never going to be vulnerable again!* Self-protection seems like a reasonable response. Unfortunately, in a sense that multiplies the harm, because it puts something you deeply care about off-limits. In addition to experiencing the pain of betrayal and loss, you also don't get to enjoy any of the benefits of loving and connecting.

It's like two sides of the same coin. One side is connection, caring, and support—put simply, love—and the other side is criticism, betrayal, and abandonment—put simply, hurt. To approach love, you have to simultaneously open yourself up to the possibility of hurt. Doing so is an act of courage. It's treating yourself as valid and whole. It's living your life in a way that matters, and it's focused on how you want to be, rather than simply whatever happens.

Let's take a closer look at this dynamic. Get an index card or small piece of scrap paper, and write down an important value on one side. On the other side, write about the possible pain that could show up if you pursue that value. Go ahead and do it now.

***

Now take a look at the card. Notice that if you throw it away, you could get rid of the possibility of pain, but you'd also be throwing away your value, and the rewards of living in alignment with that value. That's the conundrum we all face, and that's why we refer to a life well lived as vital, rather than happy. Vitality means living in a way that matters, not that everything will always turn out great. That simply isn't possible. However, if you live in a way that matters, a vital way, you'll have a full range of experiences in life, including a great deal of joy. You'll have joy *and* pain, success *and* failure, hope *and* fear.

Of course, you can focus on trying to protect yourself from the negative, but that doesn't tend to work well. Pain will creep in anyway. Plus, playing the avoidance game can create feelings of lacking purpose and even depression, which is extremely painful. So trying to shield yourself from pain can unintentionally and paradoxically create a great deal of pain.

Do you want to spend your life trying hard to avoid pain, or do you want to live boldly, choosing to act in alignment with your values and allowing both the positive and the negative to flow naturally? We can all afford to get a little more comfortable being uncomfortable. When we do, the world is full of wonders and opportunities. As always, the choice is yours, and it's always available to you.

Going Further

Living your values takes practice. You can't identify them once and be done with it. It's like navigating with a compass: you need to check back in periodically. Maybe you've drifted a bit and are no longer traveling east. Or perhaps your values have changed, or the priority of some of your values has changed. That's perfectly okay. But if you don't check in, you won't be clear about where you're going and whether you might want to make a course correction. As with everything in this book, the key is practice, practice, practice! The rest of this chapter provides exercises that will help you practice and persist in values-based living.

EXTENDED PRACTICE EXERCISE: Reminding Yourself of Your Values

This is the simplest exercise we have in the book. How can you keep your values in focus when it's so easy to get lost in the details and seemingly narrow and repetitive day-to-day tasks? How about a values reminder? Identify an object that can help remind you of something important to you. For example, if being active, healthy, and engaged with your grandkids is important to you, put a picture of your grandkids where you'll see it as you cook to remind you why healthy choices are about more than following a diet. Or if being loving and supportive toward family members is important to you, try posting a small phrase that's meaningful to you on your computer or somewhere you'll see it often as a reminder of how you want to behave. You could also choose to wear something special, such as a bracelet, to symbolize an important value. Pick three values reminders and use them to help you orient to your values each day.

EXTENDED PRACTICE EXERCISE: Assessing Whether Your Values Have Changed

We've discussed how a narrow focus on weight and dieting rules can actually hurt your chances of succeeding in weight loss. One way that can happen is if you have the thought *I screwed up*. That thought is often followed by some version of *Screw it!* (thanks, mind!), followed by unhealthful food choices or bingeing. The logic is simple: *Since I messed up and ate too many calories, I've blown my diet, so it doesn't matter if I keep eating.* Popular diet advice is to try to avoid that kind of all-or-nothing thinking. That sounds good in theory, but as you've learned, your mind is going to do what it does, and you don't have much say in the matter.

We propose a different approach to this trap: Check in with your values. When you get off course, ask yourself whether your values have changed. In most cases the answer will be no. And here's the beauty of values-based living: If you do something that isn't consistent with your values, like eat a huge piece of cake when you didn't plan to, you can immediately turn around and do things that are consistent with your values, like prepare a healthy meal for the next day, exercise, give the rest of the cake to a neighbor, and so on. The moment you engage in values-consistent behavior, you're back on track. You don't have to wait for the pounds to come off again; you've righted the ship.

The trick is to quickly reorient to your values and start doing values-consistent behaviors. That way you'll gain less weight in the short term and continue to lose more weight in the long term because you sidestepped what might be called the screw-it trap. You aren't measuring your life with calories (especially not calories you've already consumed); you're measuring your life with your actions and what you're doing in the moment. And you can always choose to live according to your values in each new moment.

Practice this approach for a month. Every time you notice that you've gotten off track with your eating, notice the pull of *Screw it!* When you notice it, stop whatever you're doing and take a few moments to write about your health values and what's important to you. Come up with three behaviors consistent with your health values that you can do that day, preferably in that moment or right away. Then make a commitment to do those three things. Here's an example of how you might format that in your journal.

Situation: *Had three pieces of pizza at a party at work.*

What did your mind say? *"I'm a failure. I never lose weight. I'm weak."*

What did you feel? *Hopeless, sad, and shameful.*

What are your health values? *To be active and engaged, to nourish my body, to build energy for my relationships and personal interests.*

What can you do today? *I can take a long walk. I can make a healthy meal plan for the next three days. I can ask a friend for support in making healthful food choices for the rest of the week.*

Remember to do this for at least one month. This practice will go a long way toward building new habits that are healthier and more consistent with your values.

EXTENDED PRACTICE EXERCISE: Negotiating Values Conflicts

Clients often tell us, "I can't do everything. What should I do when my values conflict with each other?" In this situation, the first thing to notice is that the mind has entered the equation. It tends to set up false conflicts that seem to require an all-or-nothing, black-or-white answer. Typically, however, this approach isn't relevant to values-based living.

Let's say you value being a productive, engaged worker and also being a loving, caring family member. Sometimes you might notice that work demands seem to prevent you from living up to your value in regard to family. However, the question here isn't which value you should focus on; it's how you can live your values within the practical constraints of your life. In other words, if you aren't home as much as you'd like to be, how can you stay connected? Can you send a quick, loving e-mail? Can you bring home a sign of affection, like flowers or a small gift? And more importantly, when you are home, how can you spend that time well? What if you skipped a TV show in favor of a long chat or helped with something in the limited time you had? What if you took your partner on a date? Even in the most difficult situations, such as one person working the night shift and the other working days, you can still spend whatever waking hours you have together in a loving, caring way if you connect to your values and identify behaviors consistent with those values. The key isn't which value you should focus on, but how you can behave consistently with your values with the limited time and resources available to you.

With health-related values, a common complaint is not having time to be active. But the time is actually often there if people choose to use it that way. Your mind may have given you rules about how long you must exercise: *You must work out for at least thirty minutes or it's not worth it.* Hogwash! Even ten minutes of exercise will be beneficial. And if you work out for ten minutes three times a day, you're up to thirty minutes.

The human mind is a master at creating values conflicts. Make sure you recognize when that's happening, and then reorient to what you can do given the time and resources available to you.

Right now, try to identify at least two areas where you seem to have values conflicts. In your journal, write the heading "Values Conflicts" and then list them. For each, write about how you can live that value within any practical constraints you face. Brainstorm five to ten ways you can live each value, and be sure to include both small and somewhat larger actions. Then make a plan for trying some of those options over the next week. At the end of the week, be sure to review your plan to see whether you did everything you intended. If you didn't, try again the next week or choose other values-consistent actions that might be a better fit for your life at this time. If you did accomplish those actions, reassess whether you still seem to have a values conflict, and if you do, choose more actions to try over the next week.

EXTENDED PRACTICE EXERCISE: Reclaiming Joy in Physical Activity

Your body is always there for you, and often it works in silence. How can you use activities to show gratitude to your body? Physical activity can provide a sense of purpose and is in many ways a loving act. It initiates processes in the brain that enhance the production of neurotransmitters that foster well-being. Of course, it also strengthens the heart and boosts blood circulation.

Exercise can take various forms, such as lifting weights, walking, fitness classes, dancing, swimming, and yoga. It can also simply be physical activity, such as climbing stairs, gardening, or housecleaning. Think about physical activities you could do that would embody self-care and health for you. Maybe you want to develop more strength, create more harmony and balance in your body, or foster a sense of being present in your body.

In your journal, write the heading "Physical Activities I Want to Try," and then list as many activities as you can. Feel free to search the Internet or brainstorm with other people. Go ahead and write your list now.

***

Over the next six to eight weeks, commit to engaging in at least three of these activities regularly. When you do, make sure you give them an honest effort at least four or five times before evaluating them. In the long run, it's crucial that you choose activities that you enjoy so you'll continue doing them. If you don't find much immediate enjoyment in exercise, try to identify other benefits, such as how they can foster qualities that you'd like to develop. Over time, note the overall changes in your energy level and physical functioning, along with any other benefits.

EXTENDED PRACTICE EXERCISE: Reclaiming the Joy of Healthy Eating

Your body is nourished and healed by healthful foods. Consuming nutrient-dense, fiber-rich whole foods helps make sure your body functions optimally and reduces the chance of illness and disease while also providing energy that allows you to live in bold, vital ways. The staples of a healthful diet are fruits, vegetables, whole grains, legumes (beans and peas), nuts, and seeds, along with limited amounts of fish, lean meat, and dairy products, if you choose to eat them. Most people eat less of these healthy foods than is optimal—often much less. This exercise is designed to help you reclaim the joy of eating these healthful foods.

In your journal, write the heading "Healthy Recipes I Want to Try." Then spend a little time each day searching the Internet or cookbooks for healthful recipes that include a lot of fruits, vegetables, whole grains, or legumes. You can also ask other people for recipe recommendations. Commit to trying one new recipe each week and building up your collection of healthful recipes. If you find a dish enjoyable or satisfying, look for others like it. Keep the ones you like on file, and keep trying new ones for at least eight weeks As you integrate more healthy foods into your diet, note any changes in your energy level and physical functioning, and see if those fit with your values.

Summary

This chapter was about clarifying your values, knowing what's important to you, and taking action, in the present moment to live in alignment with your values. We believe that you will find joy in healthy habits like moving your body, eating nutritious food, fostering relationships, extending compassion and gratitude toward yourself, and engaging in activities that are meaningful to you. Values can be your compass in pursuing what matters to you most, helping you plot a course of desired behaviors, giving you the strength to persist in the face of difficulties, and opening up opportunities to do new things or things that had seemed off-limits. You can choose to act with willingness and live in alignment with your values in any moment. Values-based living is an approach that will enrich your life.

CHAPTER 6

Putting It All Together

Lisa started gaining weight after her son died. Living with that unimaginable pain, she found comfort in food. During grief therapy, she began to open up to her sadness and make room for it as a part of her life. She also became more aware of and accepting of her thoughts and stopped fighting them. Her thoughts, after all, were tied to the memory of her son, and getting rid of thoughts of him would mean losing so many wonderful memories of him.

As Lisa developed more acceptance, she also changed her relationship to food and started using it more for nourishment and less for comfort. In addition, she became more engaged with her grandchildren, in keeping with her value of wanting to have a positive influence on them. She started exercising and began connecting with the people she loved more often and more deeply. And as she increasingly connected with what was important in her life and brought her behavior more in line with her values, she lost weight. In short, she was a great success.

However, she also found that life had other tests in store for her. Her husband lost his job, and for the first time in years they were in financial trouble. The stress drove her back to eating for comfort, and she began to gain weight again. She also started to once again become more disengaged from the people she cared about.

In some ways, Lisa's experience is common. People who are able to establish new healthy habits often have difficulty maintaining those habits. Life has a way of sending new stressors our way, and this often increases our contact with familiar friends in the form of unwanted thoughts and feelings.

Full Speed Ahead

You've certainly come a long way, and we're so happy that you've stuck with us on this journey! In this chapter you'll learn how to use all this book's skills together—and how to tell whether you're on track and living a values-based live or veering off course. The exercises in this chapter will help you establish new healthy habits and also return to healthy living when you face new challenges.

EXERCISE: Writing a New Life Story

In this exercise, you'll take what you've learned in this book and write a new life story for yourself with an organizing metaphor. You're the hero of this story, and you'll encounter challenges along the way. First, give this story a title that's meaningful to you. If you want to find or rediscover the joy in healthy living, perhaps your story's title would be "Loving Living." If you want to step up more boldly to the challenges of healthy living, then maybe your story's name would be "The Compassionate Challenger." Be creative and choose something that fits your experience. Open your journal and write that title on a new page. Also give your hero a name (if it's also your story's title, that's fine). This is a long exercise. Feel free to take breaks or do it over the course of a few days.

Act 1: A New Direction

In act 1, the hero wants to go in a new direction. Consult your values compass and chart a new direction of travel that will take you in a meaningful, vital direction. Draw the path in your journal and label it "Compassionate Healthy Living." You might want to extend the drawing across two pages so you have more room.

Next, draw signs along the path with messages that will let you know whether you're on track. Refer back to your work with values in chapter 5, if need be. Start with health, and then work your way through the other three domains: relationships, work or education, and personal interests. For example, signs along the path might be for exercising, preparing healthy lunches at home, educating yourself about food, or eating lots of vegetables. For relationships, signs might be things like engaging in activities with family members, being kind to your children, listening compassionately to friends, or being intimate with your partner. You can draw different paths for the different areas of life, if that helps. As you see these signs again and again, you know you're heading in the direction you want to go. You're living the new story of you. If you're no longer passing those signs, you might be off track. That's a sign too: a sign that you need to check and see what led you astray.

Act 2: Conflict

On your adventure, you encounter many mischief makers. They get you off track by telling you to do things that are inconsistent with compassionate, healthy living. You know these mischief makers well. They are your unwanted thoughts, feelings, and bodily sensations, such as cravings or fatigue. Give your recurring thoughts, feelings, and sensations names: Captain Chocolate Craving, Super Stress Man, the Indulgence Monster, Too Busy Tommy, Professor Party Time, Mr. I Can't, Shameful Sally, Nervous Ned, and so on. Identify your five most familiar mischief makers and list them in your journal, making sure you have at least one of each type (thoughts, feelings, and sensations).

Then create a personality for each of the five. For example, Captain Chocolate Craving is a dapper and convincing fellow who always shows up when the hero is most vulnerable. Mr. I Can't is matter-of-fact. He's always sure of himself and constantly tells the hero what he or she *can't* do. Review what you wrote in your journal when working through chapters 2, 3, and 4 to flesh out an identity for each character. What kinds of things do they say? How do they act?

Next, write a brief story about how the hero used to react to each mischief maker. What were the hero's old habits? When the hero tried to fight each mischief maker, what happened? What did the hero eventually do to appease each mischief maker and get it to ease up? Also explore whether this got the hero off track in terms of values-based living. Detail any unhealthy avoidance behaviors that opted for short-term comfort at the expense of valued living in the long run.

Also consider this: Are these mischief makers really out to hurt the hero? Does Shameful Sally want the hero to feel pain just because she's evil? Is Super Stress Man just screwing with the hero? Or, like the misguided motivational speaker from chapter 3, do these seeming obstructionists, these thoughts, feelings, and bodily sensations, actually have good intentions, if misguided? Are they possibly, even if in an unhelpful way, trying to protect the hero from harm? For example, maybe Shameful Sally remembers times when you were hurt badly and doesn't want you to feel that way again. She's actually looking out for you. Maybe Super Stress Man wants you to be the best you can be and worries that you can't handle it all. Maybe Captain Chocolate Craving remembers when chocolate was the one thing that could help you feel better.

In a strange way, these mischief makers do have good intentions. But when your life changes, as it will, they don't keep up. Eating chocolate to feel good doesn't work when you want to improve your health. Avoiding intimacy to appease Shameful Sally creates emptiness in your relationship.

It's like you need to write a letter, but your mind is handing you a hammer, not a pen. A hammer is a useful tool, but it's inappropriate for the job at hand. The mischief makers are well-meaning. They want to protect you and help you survive, but they're the wrong tools for the job, and they're getting in the way.

See if you can find the good intentions behind the unhelpful approach of each of your mischief makers, then write those intentions in each personality profile.

Act 3: Resolution

As the adventure progresses, the hero is able to recognize the good, if misguided, intentions that motivate each mischief maker. This allows the hero to use kindness and compassion to acknowledge the mischief makers and relate to them differently. Instead of arguing with and trying to defeat them, the hero invites them to come along on the journey, despite the distraction they can be. The key is that the hero keeps moving along the path, no matter how large, noisy, or distracting the group of mischief makers is.

Think about the five mischief makers you've been describing, and write about how the hero could respond to each in a kind, self-compassionate, and effective way in order to keep moving along the path. Again, you may want to refer back to your work in chapters 2 through 4. For example, consider an encounter with Too Busy Tommy. Instead of arguing with him, the hero acknowledges that Tommy will always feel too busy, and that it's okay if Tommy walks with the hero and screams, *Too busy!* the whole way. Or the hero might encounter Shameful Sally and, instead of trying to banish her, acknowledge her and honor the pain she's been through, standing with her as together they boldly pursue the things that matter, like going to the beach, working out, or dancing. Write a story about how the hero treats each mischief maker with loving-kindness and invites each along on the journey.

The mischief makers may have looked scary in the beginning, but now they probably seem a bit like the seven dwarfs. They can be annoying and persistent, but they are actually well-meaning. It's okay if they accompany you on the trip. In fact, sometimes those mischief makers can be darn helpful. The fact that they show up could be a signal that you have an opportunity for growth.

Imagine that you've consistently been eating foods that are nourishing and promote weight loss, and then you attend a party with a huge spread of delicious food. Immediately, you notice that the Indulgence Monster jumps out from a dark alley right into your path. If you notice this, you have a chance to resolve the conflict by doing something different, by engaging this mischief maker with kindness and self-compassion and continuing to pursue what matters to you: compassionate, healthy living. Even though the Indulgence Monster badly wants you to enjoy everything that's available, you can let him be there and still make healthy choices with your behavior.

Circling Back

At times you *will* find yourself off track. The first and easiest solution is to simply see if you lost track of your intended direction. For example, maybe you had an unusually busy week and you ate out more than you intended and didn't exercise. If so, don't beat yourself up. Instead, gently reorient to your values, set some goals, and be on your way.

If certain mischief makers continue to get in the way, it may be helpful to review the earlier chapters. The most common mischief makers are unhelpful thoughts (self-sabotaging and judgmental thoughts, reasons, and rules), uncomfortable emotions (feeling sad, anxious, stressed, deprived, bored, and so on), and cravings.

If you find yourself struggling with unhelpful thoughts, go back to chapter 3. Review the strategies and practice the exercises (or, if you've zipped through this book, try doing some of them for the first time). Become more mindfully aware of your thoughts and practice strategies to help you step back from them. Work on seeing them simply as thoughts, rather than absolute truths. Watch your thoughts, recognize their automatic and often random nature, thank your mind for them, and then, with self-compassion, move back to the business of living. Basically, notice the mischief makers for what they are—unhelpful thoughts—and let them be. Your job is to treat them with kindness and invite them along as you continue on your path.

If you find yourself trying to avoid or fix uncomfortable feelings or cravings, go back to chapter 4. See the good if misguided intentions that motivate your mischief makers. Then smile at your mischief makers, open up to them, and open up around them. Pull apart each experience into its components, one by one, and just sit with the experience and make room for it. Review what acting with willingness means, and practice some of the exercises again. Set some new goals that will help you live your values in the presence of discomfort so you can practice acting with willingness. It's important to practice living your values in both easy and difficult situations. That's where the vitality of living well really arises. Living your values even in the face of difficulties is courageous. Approaching your feelings with kindness and self-compassion is the work of a hero.

All's Well That Lives Well

You've assuredly heard the phrase "All's well that ends well." Here's how that might be translated: "As long as everything goes the way I want, I'm cool. I don't care how we got there." We invite you to take a different stance toward your life. How about "All's well that *lives* well"? Why "lives well"? Because that's the part you can control: what you do and how you live. From our perspective, if you act with willingness, if you invite the mischief makers of fear, anxiety, sadness, doubt, and judgment along on the journey and really do what matters to you...things won't always go well. What?! That's right, we said things won't always go well. Sometimes everything will go wonderfully, and other times life will feel like a disaster.

Life is unpredictable, and you can't control what other people do. So what you're left with is how *you* want to be as a person in each and every moment of your life. You can be loving despite receiving anger back, because being loving is important to you. You can go to a party and connect with friends even if people make comments about you eating or not eating, because connecting is one of your values. You can be intimate even if your partner rejects you, because fostering intimacy is deeply important to you. You can go dancing even though your mind tells you how awful you look, because dancing is something you care about doing.

No matter what the outcome, there's vitality in living your values. You stay true to yourself and grow, even as you're deeply challenged. From now on, direct your focus to what you're doing, rather than what's happening to you. Give yourself credit for what you *can* control: your behavior. Strive to be everything you've ever wanted to be. Live your life boldly!

How to Stay on Course

Like most people (us included), you may find that you get in a groove and then forget about some of the unhelpful traits of your mind—the world's worst motivational speaker, and the source of all mischief makers, unhelpful rules and reasons, and sticky thoughts. The next thing you know, *bam!* You've fallen into the fix-me trap. In the sections that follow, we offer several helpful tips that can help you stay the course or navigate back to your intended path when your mind has led you off course.

Pounds Versus Living

We want to share a secret with you: healthy living often actually does feel good. It can also lead to at least temporary improvements in self-confidence. This is fine. After all, feeling good, well, feels good. There's nothing wrong with that. But sometimes your mind may take over and start telling you, *I feel good. My thoughts are good… I must be fixed! The fix-me agenda really works!* As we've emphasized, a vital life includes a wide range of thoughts and feelings. When those are mostly good, it's fine to enjoy the experience, but be careful not to confuse feeling good with living well.

The number one place we see this show up with clients is with the scale. When you're losing weight, the scale can be a constant source of validation. The pounds keep going down, and you keep feeling better. It can be easy to forget that this is about compassionate, healthy living. The problem is, when the number on the scale stops going down, you're left with a feeling of emptiness, after which difficult thoughts and feelings return. But thoughts and feelings don't provide useful guidance for behavior. Values do.

Cheating

We'll put this bluntly: There's no cheating in compassionate, healthy living! Cheating doesn't even enter the equation. True cheating goes something like this: You lie on your income tax return, the government gets less tax revenue, and that means less revenue for government spending and programs. "Cheating" on your diet isn't cheating at all. It's simply a behavior, an act. Nobody is cheated out of anything, nobody is there to pass judgment, and nobody loses. Your mind will tell you that you're cheating; that's something minds do. What's really going on is that you aren't living consistently with your values. When you remove "should," "must," and "cheat" from the equation, you're left with just you and what you want to be about.

The Perfection Trap

The idea that if you aren't perfect, you've failed, is another offering from the ever-helpful mind. If you notice a constant internal chatter characterized by self-criticism, focusing on what you didn't do rather than what you did, you can be pretty sure the world's worst motivational speaker is at work.

This can even show up with values. Your mind may tell you that you aren't doing enough or that you could be doing better. Of course, sometimes it's useful to see if you can make adjustments to get your life more in line with your values. But be careful here. For every time it might be useful to reevaluate your priorities, there might be five, ten, or one hundred times when your mind is just criticizing you. If you stop moving along your path to struggle with that critical mischief maker each time those thoughts show up, that's going to get in the way of doing important things. Often, the best move is to reorient to what you can do in that moment, that day, or that week to get moving again. Just let the criticism come along for the ride—and know that sometimes it will be very loud!

Barriers to Growth

You may find that you're living a more values-driven life, and suddenly some new mischief maker shows up. A classic one is when your mind accuses you of being selfish and tells you that you don't deserve to take time for yourself—that you need to spend that time doing things for others.

165

Bear in mind that there are both short-term and long-term effects of almost any action. Let's look at the example of going for a walk when your family would rather you stayed at home. In the short term, your family might be unhappy that you're doing something for yourself. A family member might even say something upsetting or complain that you didn't do a chore or task that would have been helpful.

But assuming you're taking care of your basic responsibilities in regard to your family, taking care of yourself will almost always help you be more engaged, connected, and nurturing in the long run. Treating yourself with love and kindness helps you shower others with the same care. Unfortunately, your mind might not get that—ever. It might jump out and shout at you every time you're working out but could be doing something else. You might need to make room for that mischief maker on your journey.

On a related note, you might find that your partner or family members are afraid of you changing. It shouldn't work that way, but realize that they have their own set of mischief makers telling them what to do and say. As you lose weight and feel better, your partner might feel insecure or have another mischief maker pop up, getting louder and louder and shouting that you're going to start getting attention from other people or that you won't love your partner anymore.

See if you can climb behind your partner or family member's eyes. Imagine what the other person's journey feels like. Then connect to your values and act with loving-kindness, even in the face of criticism or lack of support. You can still be the person you want to be. Act with willingness, be compassionate, and live in alignment with your relationship values. Most often others will eventually come around after you reassure them through your actions.

Letting Go of Explanations

People are always explaining themselves. Whether these explanations are true or false seldom interests us. Explanations have their place, but they are often offered when the situation doesn't call for it.

People certainly don't need to be justified. Consider for a moment how much self-justification and explanation you do within yourself, as if the court-of-you will finally judge you to be innocent if your explanation of your "crimes" is good enough. In this fantasy, you will somehow walk out of the court-of-you a free person some day.

Sometimes people's actions need explanation, but more often, whether something was done or not done is all we really need to know: "I ate a cheeseburger." "I watched three hours of television." These kinds of statements, whether said aloud or just as thoughts, are almost always accompanied by "because..." Unfortunately, the explanation often becomes a trap: *If only I had been more motivated (smarter, better, kinder...). But I wasn't, and now I must accept my fate.*

Alternatively, you may carry a sense that you should be able to explain yourself but can't, and therefore feel you're somehow insufficient or a failure. That too becomes a trap: *I've failed, and there's no good reason for it. I'll never succeed.*

Among our clients, we've often seen "why" become an obsession. People can obsess about finding "proper" explanations: "I'm addicted." "I don't have enough time." "My family habits make me eat too much." "My history makes it too hard for me to open up to people." Sometimes clients are surprised at how little interest we have in their explanations or how little time we spend pursuing explanations.

What we care about is what works. We care about what small act you might engage in today that could suffuse your life with more meaning, vitality, and purpose. Explanations of why you did or didn't do something are easy to come by—and they often don't make a lot of difference. Engaging in even the smallest values-based act outweighs any explanation.

We don't mean to sound harsh. We aren't saying that explanations are necessarily untrue. Rather, it's that they obscure what's really important if you want to change your behavior. The human mind is resourceful and can explain almost anything away. Far too often, people are satisfied with a good explanation. We're much more interested in actions than explanations about actions. Did you engage in a valued activity or not? Either way, how did that work?

Your mind, ever the unhelpful mischief maker, will get quite worked up in the name of explanation and justification. That's okay. Your job is to notice that, step back from it, and focus on the one thing that truly matters: living your life.

EXTENDED PRACTICE EXERCISE: Being a Scientist

In any situation, for any reason, if you find yourself struggling, you can turn to this simple exercise. Approach whatever activity you're doing as if you were a scientist. Your one goal is to get deeply in touch with what's happening and document it for later study.

Start with your body. What sensations do you notice? Where are they? Where do they begin and end? How do they feel? Imagine you're observing these sensations for the very first time and with pure curiosity. Make note of everything you feel.

Next, observe your thoughts. What kinds of thoughts are you having? See if you can notice and categorize them: "There's a fear," "Here's a judgment," "This is a random thought about nonsense," "That's a worry about something that might happen in the future," "That's a to-do item I don't want to forget," and so on. Watch your thoughts dispassionately and categorize them without getting caught in them. Marvel at your mind's complexity, tenacity, and seeming randomness as if you're observing it for the first time.

Finally, move to your feelings. Note any feeling states and watch them as they ebb and flow. Try to feel them as though you're feeling them for the first time. Observe them in a way that's designed to study them, as if you were going to write an essay about what they feel like.

After observing all of these aspects of your experience like a scientist, check in and see what's important to you in that moment. See if you can find a small way to act with willingness in that moment and let the rest of your experience come along for the ride.

Summary

This entire book comes down to a simple choice: Will you choose to live your values, even when it's difficult or uncomfortable, and even when your mind gives you a hundred reasons you shouldn't? This is a choice you'll face often, and you always get to make that choice. Sometimes you may not see the choice, but it's there. We all get to decide what to do with our behavior. We don't get to choose how we think or feel or what the outcomes of our behavior will be, but we do get to decide what we do.

It's like a light switch: You can always chose to turn it on and pursue what's important to you. There are times when the switch will be off. There is no "should" or "have to" here. It's your life, and you can do whatever you want with it. The goal isn't to be perfect; rather, the goal is to move toward a life with more vitality, compassion, and satisfaction.

If you find yourself off track, you can always use these simple questions to get you back on course: "Am I behaving consistently with my values and goals?" "Am I buying into unhelpful thoughts?" "Am I trying to avoid feeling a certain way?"

Life is a big, messy, gorgeous, disastrous, joyful thing. Try flipping that light switch on a little more often than you already do, and just see what happens.

CHAPTER 7

Weight Loss Know-How

At its core, weight loss is simple math. To lose weight, you need to burn more calories than you take in through eating. That's really it. Of course, it can be hard to put this knowledge into practice, for many reasons. At the most basic level, it's difficult to lose weight if you don't know how to monitor the number of calories you consume versus the number you burn. You can also benefit from some simple knowledge that can help you tip that balance in your favor. This chapter will fill you in on some of the details or serve as a short refresher course.

You may wonder why in the world we put this chapter last. Isn't this what weight loss is really about? As you now know, we don't think so. Although the information in this chapter is very useful and not overly complicated, if weight loss were just a matter of education, there would be far fewer overweight people. In reality, this information gets used in ways that don't work very well. If you've fallen into a fix-me trap of trying to lose weight because you believe it will improve how you think and feel, along with most other aspects of your life, without you having to change what you do, the information in this chapter won't take you very far. If you use this information to sentence yourself to a rigid, unfulfilling diet and exercise regimen, you might see good results in the short term, but they're likely to fade over time. It's not a matter of having information; it's how you use it.

We've put this chapter at the end of the book so you can use the information in the service of a values-based, healthy life. Hopefully you'll use counting calories as a way to provide appropriate nourishment and care to your body so that you can engage in good working habits, connect with friends and family, enjoy fulfilling activities, and treat others with love and kindness. Counting calories is much more effective and meaningful when done in the service of living a vital, satisfying life, as opposed to trying to get rid of an unwanted body shape and the thoughts and feelings that go with it. So please use this information to fuel a values-driven life.

Energy Balance

Your weight is determined by the balance between the calories (or energy) you eat and the calories you expend by being active. If you eat the same number of calories as you expend, your weight will stay about the same because the calories consumed equal, or balance, the calories expended. If you want to lose weight, the best way is to both consume fewer calories and be more active.

A deficit of 3,500 calories typically results in about 1 pound of weight loss. So if you burn 3,500 more calories than you take in over any period of time, you'll probably lose about 1 pound. You can lose weight at any pace you want. Sustainable weight loss is usually achieved by losing one to two pounds per week, although you may lose more than that in the first two to eight weeks of limiting calories and increasing exercise. A moderate approach is generally best, as severe restriction of food can cause health problems. It also isn't consistent with a values-driven life. We don't endorse extreme, unsustainable diets.

Here's a rough guideline regarding how many calories you should be consuming, in both foods and beverages, to lose 1 to 2 pounds per week based on your current weight, though you may need more if you're very active:

If you weigh less than 200 pounds, aim for about 1,200 calories per day.

If you weigh 200 to 300 pounds, aim for about 1,500 calories per day.

If you weigh more than 300 pounds, aim for about 1,800 calories per day.

If you're overweight, losing just 10 percent of your body weight will result in significant health benefits, including lower blood pressure and cholesterol levels. So if you weigh 190 pounds, and weight loss is a part of compassionate, healthy living for you, losing 19 pounds is a good first goal. Losing that amount of weight and maintaining the weight loss will provide significant health benefits over time.

EXERCISE: Calculating How Many Calories You Typically Burn

Now it's time to test your math skills. (Sorry!) In your journal, write "A: Resting metabolic rate" on one line, "B: Calories burned by day-to-day activities" on the next, and "C: Calories burned by exercise" on a third. Then go to a website where you can calculate your resting metabolic rate (for example, http://www.bmi-calculator.net/bmr-calculator). This is the number of calories you burn simply by being alive. In other words, if you stayed in bed all day, you'd burn this many calories. You'd also probably be pretty bored, but we digress. Write that number on line A in your journal.

We all engage in daily activities, such as climbing stairs, doing household chores, and moving around from one place to another. These activities also burn calories. A good estimate is 350 calories if you're fairly sedentary, and 550 if you're fairly active, for example, being on your feet a lot, having to walk around for your job, or doing lots of housework, gardening, or lawn care. Write that number on line B in your journal.

If you do physical activity for the purpose of exercise, that also burns calories. Those calories go on line C. If you're fairly active (exercising for about twenty to thirty minutes per day on average), that probably burns between 100 and 150 calories. If you don't engage in any activity for exercise, leave line C blank. If your activity level is moderate, falling somewhere in between, that probably burns 50 to 75 calories. Once you've filled in line C, add the three numbers.

Here's an example for a forty-five-year-old woman who is five foot four and weighs 190 pounds:

A:	1,571
B:	350
C:	50
Total:	1,971

This woman burns about 1,971 calories per day. Knowing that it takes a deficit of 3,500 calories to produce 1 pound of weight loss, and knowing that losing 1 to 2 pounds per week is sustainable, a good goal for this woman would be to consume 1,200 to 1,400 calories per day. That would produce a deficit of 570 to 770 calories per day, so she would lose a pound every five to seven days.

Voilà! You are now a weight loss expert. Wait, you want to know more? Okay, let's talk about food.

Food

There are no specific foods you have to eat and or not eat as long as you balance calories consumed and burned. However, do use reasonable judgment. You know that eating 1,200 calories of doughnuts isn't healthy. The best approach is to eat healthful whole foods that you'll continue eating after losing weight. Work on including more healthy foods that you like or can develop a taste for in your diet.

Whole grains, vegetables, legumes, and fruits are the healthiest foods you can eat. They contain a lot of nutrients, and many studies show that they help the body function better and promote long-term health (Block, Patterson, and Subar 1992; Sacks et al. 2001). This information is nothing new, but it bears repeating: Avoid processed and packaged food as much as possible. Look for natural ingredients. And, when possible, buy whole foods and make your own meals.

These healthful foods provide another key benefit. Many of them are nutrient-dense and low in calories. That means you can eat larger portions of them, which is satisfying, while keeping the calorie balance in your favor. One very interesting study showed that people tend to eat the same weight of food, no matter what kind of food it was (Bell et al. 1998). In other words, you're likely to eat the same amount of food *by weight*, whether you sit down to a meal of steak and potatoes, or one of salad, brown rice, veggies, and some lean protein, such as turkey. However the second meal is lower in calories, so there are fewer to burn later. It's also higher in nutrients and provides many health benefits.

You may think you don't like vegetables. Most people who think this haven't experimented much with preparation methods, seasonings, or combinations of vegetables. Commit to eating more vegetables, and to trying lots of recipes and making it fun. Also, be aware that food preferences can change—if you give them a chance to. You need to limit your intake of high-fat, high-sugar foods, like soda, cake, cookies, and the like. Otherwise you'll have a harder time changing your food preferences.

In general, a lower-fat diet does help people lose weight (Tuomilehto et al. 2001; Look AHEAD Research Group 2007). However, calories are the most important factor. If you eat all low-fat and nonfat items but consume 2,500 calories per day, you won't lose weight unless you're extremely active. We hate to break it to you, but that low-fat cheese isn't a healthy option if you consume a lot of it. Ultimately, you need to look at how specific foods fit into your overall diet. You must have a calorie deficit to lose weight, regardless of what foods you eat. That said, because reducing fat intake has been associated with positive health benefits (Knowler et al. 2002), it's often recommended. Limiting sugar has also been associated with better health (Lustig, Schmidt, and Brindis 2012).

Be aware that severely restricting your consumption of desired foods can backfire. If you feel deprived, those foods may seem to gain more allure. You may have noticed this. Have you ever sworn off certain foods only to later find yourself consuming them compulsively? If you love ice cream, don't cut it out completely, just have it less frequently, perhaps once or twice a month as a treat. And when you do have it, fit it in by forgoing calories from other foods. In other words, plan and prepare for the occasional indulgence.

Balancing Nutrition and Pleasure

Think of the food you eat as having two attributes: pleasure and nutrition. The key is finding foods that are pack a nutritional punch while also providing pleasure. For example, many people find sweet potatoes, red bell peppers, and salad—all foods with high nutritional value—to be fairly pleasurable. Aim to get the majority of the food you eat from this high-pleasure, high-nutrition category. Cake, cookies, and most desserts are tend to be high on pleasure but low on nutrition, but they have a place too. You want a limited amount of the food you eat to come from this high-pleasure, low-nutrition category so you don't feel too deprived. If you tend to be a picky eater, it's important that you also include foods in the low-pleasure, high-nutrition category. Maybe for you this is broccoli, kale, or Brussels sprouts. (By the way, we love Brussels sprouts and encourage you to give them a chance!)

Finally, there's the low-pleasure, low-nutrition category. This is the one case where we encourage avoidance! This category usually comes into play when you're at a social gathering or eating out, or when a family member keeps unhealthy snacks around that you don't like very much. For example, say you aren't a fan of key lime pie or you're not fond of things made with mayonnaise, but you have some because that's what's being served or just what's around. That's a lose-lose proposition. There's no reason to waste calories on something you won't even get much pleasure from. Try making long lists of foods that fall into each of the four categories and using them to guide your choices.

Mindful Eating

Eating is something we can do on automatic pilot, so it's not surprising that we often direct our attention elsewhere. Many of us eat in front of the TV, on the go, or at our desks. However, when you eat while distracted, it's hard to make a memory of what you ate. Your brain is occupied, and it isn't taking in all the relevant information. Without that information, we tend to overeat and, perhaps worse, default to thinking we need a big meal later.

You can counteract this with a few simple strategies. Start by eating in a designated area. If you don't already do so, sit at your dining table or in the break room at work, as opposed to on the couch or at your desk. Pause before you eat and become aware of everything on your plate for just five seconds.

Eat slowly, putting your utensils down after each bite. Pay attention to all aspects of the food: its appearance, aromas, textures, and flavors. It's amazing how often we don't actually taste the food we eat. Also practice being mindful of what the food will do for you and your body, whether it will provide useful, sustained energy for your body, and how you'll use that energy to fuel a values-driven life.

Keeping Track

Without a doubt, the single most powerful thing you can do to help yourself lose weight is record what you consume. Writing everything down as you eat it or drink it, along with the number of calories, and then adding up the total number of calories consumed daily has been proven helpful in losing weight and keeping it off (Baker and Kirschenbaum 1993; Wing and Hill 2001). It may be obvious why, but we'll say it anyway: If you don't know exactly what's going into your body, there's no way to know if you're in a calorie deficit. There are online helpful tracking tools (for example, at http://myfitnesspal.com), or you can simply keep a written journal in a small notebook, using one page for each day. You can also track fat or protein consumption, but it isn't necessary. The key is to make it a habit you'll continue to do. Tracking food and calories consumed will help you lose weight.

You'll also need a guide to calories in different foods. There are many helpful tools online, or you can buy a book that provides this information, such as *The CalorieKing Calorie, Fat, and Carbohydrate Counter*, by Allan Borushek. Tracking calories can be laborious at first. We won't sugarcoat it: It's a pain in the butt looking up everything you eat, but over time it becomes a bit easier. And if you keep a food diary as part of a values-driven life, you're doing it because it's important for your health, relationships, work, and recreational life, and each and every time you record what you've consumed, you can remain conscious of that. It matters. If, on the other hand, you do it because you're trying to fix something that's "wrong' with you, it may be a lot more like a chore.

The other tool available to you is the Nutrition Facts section on packaged food labels. Be aware that the calories and fat listed on the label are for *one* serving. To figure out how many calories you ate, you need to know if you ate the actual serving size, more, or less. Most people tend to eat more than a serving (we know we do!), so be sure to note the serving size listed on the label. If you need help interpreting the nutritional information on labels, review the Food and Drug Administration's information regarding food labels. It's available on their website (http://www.fda .gov/Food/ResourcesForYou/Consumers), under Food Facts for Consumers.

Virtually everyone underestimates their calorie intake (Heitmann and Lissner 1995; Mertz et al. 1991). Why is it so hard to be accurate? People have a natural tendency to give themselves leeway when estimating portion size or the ingredients in prepared foods, for example, when eating something at a party or restaurant. It's also typical to forget some items or intentionally omit others. It's not that people are deliberately deceiving themselves; it's just a natural tendency, compounded by living busy lives. It's best to assume that you're underrecording at all times, probably by at least 15 percent.

Measuring cups and a food scale will go a long way toward ensuring greater accuracy. For foods you eat regularly, measure out your typical portion size and see how much food it really is. If it's a packaged food, figure out how many servings you usually eat. You may get better at this over time, but there's really no substitute for simply measuring and weighing to make sure you're achieving your calorie goal. Even when you think, *I've got this*, it can be extremely helpful to start measuring again. You may find that you've drifted.

Weighing Yourself

Ultimately, the scale will tell you if you've drifted. If you think your deficit is 300 to 500 calories per day but you're steadily gaining weight, your calorie tracking is off. Try weighing and measuring all of your food for a week to see what's happening.

You may wonder how often you should weigh yourself. There's no rule, but many experts recommend no less than once per week and no more than once per day. If you weigh yourself more frequently than that you'll see fluctuations that aren't very useful. But looking at your weight over the course of a week or a month is very helpful if you use the numbers as information, not an indictment, and make any needed adjustments. Regardless of how often you weigh yourself, the best time is in the morning, right after you wake up and before you eat or drink. That will give you more consistent readings.

Physical Activity

Regular exercise helps promote weight loss because it causes you to expend more calories. For example, walking a mile burns about 100 to 200 calories, depending on your body weight and how fast you walk. However, exercise is no substitute for calorie control if your goal is weight loss. For example, you can undo three miles of walking by eating one large chocolate cookie from the bakery. Yikes! Let's not even get into ice cream or pie.

Exercise has many other benefits. It helps reduce your risk of heart disease, diabetes, and cancer, and that's true even if your weight doesn't change (Haskell et al. 2007). Being physically fit is so important for your health, no matter what you weigh. That alone should provide some good incentive to get your feet moving. Of course, regular exercise is also strongly connected to maintaining a more healthy weight.

Exercise as much as you can given the time available to you and without risking injury. If you haven't been exercising, start with something moderate, like walking, and start slow. You might try for just 25 minutes for the entire first week, and then add 25 more minutes each week. Spread it out over three days at the beginning, and then over five days as you get up to 100 minutes of exercise per week. The American College of Sports medicine recommends 250 minutes of exercise per week. Don't worry; it's fine to get there gradually.

As to what type of exercise you should do, the answer is simple: something you like! There are so many options: walking, swimming, tennis, cycling, fitness classes, exercise videos, and more. Just make sure it's cardiovascular, or aerobic. In other words, it should be something that gets your heart rate up. Generally speaking, you should be breathing fast enough that you can talk but not sing. You should be able to have a conversation with a friend while walking, but if you can break into song, speed it up! If, on the other hand, you have trouble breathing or can't talk at all, slow down.

Some people find one kind of exercise they love (or can tolerate) and just keep doing that over and over. If that works, do it. Other people need to switch things up. If you think you don't like any kind of exercise, our recommendation is to try a lot of different things. You're bound to find something you're willing to do. If time is an issue, exercise in the morning before your day gets crazy. Schedule exercise like you would a meeting that you can't miss.

Don't try to substitute everyday activities for exercise. Gardening and housecleaning are great, and you do burn calories doing those activities. However, they don't provide the health and weight benefits described above. There's no substitute for the real thing.

Also, please be safe. Before starting a new exercise program, check with your doctor to see if you have any health restrictions. To prevent injury, start any activity at a lower intensity for the first five minutes, and end each activity the same way. If you have chest pain, stop and sit down or lie down. If it doesn't go away quickly, go to an emergency room. If it does go away but returns each time you're active, see your doctor. Other exercise-related symptoms you should report to your doctor include shortness of breath, excessive sweating, light-headedness, or feeling sick to your stomach.

Set Yourself Up for Success

You can make living a healthy lifestyle easier with some simple adjustments to your home environment. Keep healthy foods and snacks in the house and in sight, and get tempting, high-calorie snacks and foods out of the house. You're much less likely to eat unhealthy foods if they aren't readily available.

Plan your meals in advance, before going to the grocery store. Make a list so you know what to buy—then buy only what's on your list. Prepare healthful foods in advance. Put healthy snacks in clear containers so you can easily see them in the cupboard or refrigerator. This makes it easier for you to make a healthy choice. Take healthy homemade lunches and snacks to work or school.

Eat out as little as possible. Restaurant meals are a major source of calories for most people. Restaurants generally try to make food taste as good as possible with little or no attention to healthfulness, and their portion sizes tend to be two to five times what's recommended. When eating out, check restaurant menus online before you go, if possible. Ask restaurants for nutrition information about their offerings, such as ingredients and calorie counts, if available. Also ask for modifications, like leaving out butter or oil, or serving dressing on the side. Restaurants are often happy to oblige. You are paying for the food, after all!

If you eat out and think you ordered an extremely healthy meal, assume it's 1,000 calories. That's right, 1,000. If you think you just got a "normal" meal, assume 2,000 calories. If you think you ate a pretty big and unhealthy meal, estimate 3,000 to 3,500 calories. If that sounds crazy, look up your favorite chain restaurant online and check the calorie content of a meal that includes a main dish, a shared appetizer, and, if you usually have one, a dessert. You'll never look at restaurant food the same again. Here's the calorie content of a "reasonable" meal at an establishment that we won't name: half of an appetizer of nachos (765 calories), salad with grilled chicken (850 calories), and half a dessert (645 calories). That's 2,260 calories! Throw in an alcoholic beverage and that's way more than a day's worth of food in one meal. The bottom line? You can't eat out regularly and lose weight.

Summary

We just gave you a lot of "rules" for losing weight. But hopefully you've learned that if following the rules isn't connected to a focus on compassionate, healthy living, it probably won't last. And you now know that losing weight to control or change how you think and feel probably isn't going to sustain your efforts in the long run. Therefore, we recommend that you use these guidelines to empower you to take positive action in your life. Nourish your body so that you can pursue a more purpose-driven, vital life. And if the "rules" aren't working—if they aren't leading you where you want to be going—throw them out. Find out what works for you and do that.

References

Baker, R. C., and D. S. Kirschenbaum. 1993. "Self-Monitoring May Be Necessary for Successful Weight Control." *Behavior Therapy* 24:377–394.

Bell, E. A., V. H. Castellanos, C. L. Pelkman, M. L. Thorwart, and B. J. Rolls. 1998. "Energy Density of Foods Affects Energy Intake in Normal-Weight Women." *American Journal of Clinical Nutrition* 67:412–420.

Block, G., B. Patterson, and A. Subar. 1992. "Fruit, Vegetables, and Cancer Prevention: A Review of the Epidemiologic Evidence." *Nutrition and Cancer: An International Journal* 18:1–29.

Borushek, A. 2012. *The CalorieKing Calorie, Fat, and Carbohydrate Counter.* Costa Mesa, CA: Family Health Publications.

Butryn, M. L., E. Forman, K. Hoffman, J. Shaw, and A. Juarascio. 2011. "A Pilot Study of Acceptance and Commitment Therapy for Promotion of Physical Activity." *Journal of Physical Activity and Health* 8:516–522.

Cramer, P., and T. Steinwert. 1998. "Thin Is Good, Fat Is Bad: How Early Does It Begin?" *Journal of Applied Developmental Psychology* 19:429–451.

Dahl, J., and T. Lundgren. 2006. *Living Beyond Your Pain: Acceptance and Commitment Therapy to Ease Chronic Pain.* Oakland, CA: New Harbinger.

French, S. A., M. Story, and R. W. Jeffery. 2001. "Environmental Influences on Eating and Physical Activity." *Annual Review of Public Health* 22:309–335.

Haskell, W. L., I. M. Lee, R. R. Pate, K. E. Powell, S. N. Blair, B. A. Franklin, et al. 2007. "Physical Activity and Public Health: Updated Recommendation for Adults from the American College of Sports Medicine and the American Heart Association." *Medicine and Science in Sports and Exercise* 39:1423–1434.

Hayes, S. C., J. B. Luoma, F. W. Bond, A. Masuda, and J. Lillis. 2006. "Acceptance and Commitment Therapy: Model, Processes, and Outcomes." *Behaviour Research and Therapy* 44:1–25.

Hayes, S. C., K. D. Strosahl, and K. G. Wilson. 1999. *Acceptance and Commitment Therapy: An Experiential Approach to Behavior Change.* New York: Guilford Press.

Hayes, S. C., K. Strosahl, K. G. Wilson, R. T. Bissett, J. Pistorello, D. Toarmino, et al. 2004. "Measuring Experiential Avoidance: A Preliminary Test of a Working Model." *Psychological Record* 54:553–578.

Heitmann, B. L., and L. Lissner. 1995. "Dietary Underreporting by Obese Individuals: Is It Specific or Non-specific?" *British Medical Journal* 311:986–989.

Hill, J. O., and J. C. Peters. 1998. "Environmental Contributions to the Obesity Epidemic." *Science* 280(5368):1371–1374.

Knowler, W. C., E. Barrett-Connor, S. E. Fowler, R. F. Hamman, J. M. Lachin, E. A. Walker, D. M. Nathan; Diabetes Prevention Program Research Group. 2002. "Reduction in the Incidence of Type 2 Diabetes with Lifestyle Intervention or Metformin." *New England Journal of Medicine* 346(6):393–403.

Lillis, J., S. C. Hayes, K. Bunting, and A. Masuda. 2009. "Teaching Acceptance and Mindfulness to Improve the Lives of the Obese: A Preliminary Test of a Theoretical Model." *Annals of Behavioral Medicine* 37:58–69.

Look AHEAD Research Group. 2007. "Reduction in Weight and Cardiovascular Disease Risk Factors in Individuals with Type 2 Diabetes: One-Year Results of the Look AHEAD Trial." *Diabetes Care* 30:1374–1383.

Lustig, R. H., L. A. Schmidt, and C. D. Brindis. 2012. "The Toxic Truth About Sugar." *Nature* 482:27–29.

Mertz, W., J. C. Tsui, J. T. Judd, S. Reiser, J. Hallfrisch, E. R. Morris, P. D. Steele, and E. Lashley. 1991. "What Are People Really Eating? The Relation Between Energy Intake Derived from Estimated Diet Records and Intake Determined to Maintain Body Weight." *American Journal of Clinical Nutrition* 54:291–295.

Puhl, R. M., and C. A. Heuer. 2009. "The Stigma of Obesity: A Review and Update." *Obesity* 17:941–964.

Puhl, R. M., and C. A. Heuer. 2010. "Obesity Stigma: Important Considerations for Public Health." *American Journal of Public Health* 100:1019 1028.

Sacks, F. M., L. P. Svetkey, W. M. Vollmer, L. J. Appel, G. A. Bray, D. Harsha, et al. 2001. "Effects on Blood Pressure of Reduced Dietary Sodium and the Dietary Approaches to Stop Hypertension (DASH) Diet." *New England Journal of Medicine* 344:3–10.

Saelens, B. E., and L. H. Epstein. 1996. "Reinforcing Value of Food in Obese and Non-obese Women." *Appetite* 27:41–50.

Schvey, N. A., R. M. Puhl, and K. D. Brownell. 2011. "The Impact of Weight Stigma on Caloric Consumption." *Obesity* 19:1957–1962.

Sheldon, K. M., and A. J. Elliot. 1998. "Not All Personal Goals Are Personal: Comparing Autonomous and Controlled Reasons for Goals as Predictors of Effort and Attainment." *Personality and Social Psychology Bulletin* 24:546–557.

Sheldon, K. M., and A. J. Elliot. 1999. "Goal Striving, Need Satisfaction, and Longitudinal Well-Being: The Self-Concordance Model." *Journal of Personality and Social Psychology* 76:482–497.

Tuomilehto, J., J. Lindstrom, J. G. Eriksson, T. T. Valle, H. Hamalainen, P. Ilanne-Parikka, et al. 2001. "Prevention of Type 2 Diabetes Mellitus by Changes in Lifestyle Among Subjects with Impaired Glucose Tolerance." *New England Journal of Medicine* 344:1343–1350.

Volkow, N. D., and R. A. Wise. 2005. "How Can Drug Addiction Help Us Understand Obesity?" *Nature Neuroscience* 8:555–560.

Walser, R. D., and D. Westrup. 2007. *Acceptance and commitment therapy for the treatment of post-traumatic stress disorder: A practitioner's guide to using mindfulness and acceptance strategies.* Oakland, CA: New Harbinger.

Wegner, D. M., D. J. Schneider, S. R. Carter, and T. L. White. 1987. "Paradoxical Effects of Thought Suppression." *Journal of Personality and Social Psychology* 53:5–13.

Wing, R. R., and J. O. Hill. 2001. "Successful Weight Loss Maintenance." *Annual Review of Nutrition* 21:323–341.

Jason Lillis, PhD, is assistant professor of research at the Alpert Medical School of Brown University and a clinical psychologist at the Miriam Hospital in Providence, RI. He is coauthor of *Acceptance and Commitment Therapy* and a leading ACT-for-weight-loss research scientist.

JoAnne Dahl, PhD, is professor of psychology at Uppsala University, Sweden. JoAnne is a clinical psychologist specializing in behavior medicine. She is coauthor of the *Art and Science of Valuing in Psychotherapy, Acceptance and Commitment Therapy for Chronic Pain, Living Beyond Your Pain, and ACT* and *RFT in Relationships.*

Sandra M. Weineland, PhD, is a clinical psychologist and doctor of psychology at Linköping University, Sweden. She is a specialist in psychotherapy. Her research has been focused on evaluating ACT for people with obesity, with the aim to help participants develop self-compassion and devote energy to living life fully and consciously.

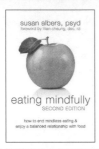
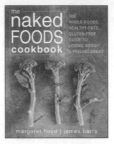
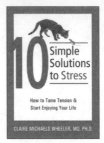
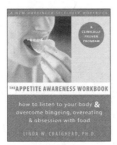
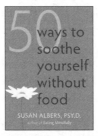
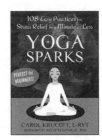